Praise for *The Vegiterranean Diet*

"We're all looking for sustainable solutions to long-term he___ ___ diet can be complicated and burdensome. Julieanna H__ ___ ___ ___ ___ ___ ___ heart of why the Mediterranean lifestyle pro__ ___ ___ ___ ___ ___ ___ccessi-ble, informing primer on the buildi__ ___ ___ ___ ___ ___ ___obust with mouth-watering plant-based rec___ ___ ___ ___ ___ ___ n and rely upon for years to come."

—___ROLL, plant-based athlete
and bestselling author of *Finding Ultra*

"Julieanna takes us on a Mediterranean journey filled with important nutritional information, debunking common food myths and providing us with a road map to a healthy lifestyle using her Vegiterranean food pyramid. This book has both educated and inspired me to live a plant-based, whole foods Vegiterranean lifestyle."

—MIKE ZIGOMANIS,
plant-based professional hockey player

"A must-read for anyone interested in a sustainable, healthy life! *The Vegiterranean Diet* brings the history and science of nutrition from antiquity into the future, offering winning arguments for a plant-based diet. Julieanna offers a very clear plan to help us change our health and change the world. I'm in!"

—LISA BLOOM, attorney and *New York Times*
bestselling author of *Think: Straight Talk for
Women to Stay Smart in a Dumbed-Down World*

"This book brings a practical and scientific perspective to the famously romantic Mediterranean diet. Julieanna is entertaining and informative as she shares everything you need to get started, from the diet's historical background, nutritional science, and impeccable health outcomes to an abundance of delicious plant-based recipes!"

—DEREK TRESIZE, CPT, WNBF Pro Bodybuilder

"A fascinating exploration into both the past and present using food and science as the vehicle, *The Vegiterranean Diet* infuses nutrition with compassion and wisdom. Julieanna Hever provides a solid and compelling thesis for why the healthiest diet is one that is plant-based, and offers an easy, delicious, and practical plan to transform your health. Viva Vegano!"

—COLLEEN PATRICK-GOUDREAU,
bestselling author of six books, including
The 30-Day Vegan Challenge and host of *Food for Thought*

"*The Vegiterranean Diet* is bursting with timely, thoughtful information. Julieanna Hever takes the Mediterranean diet to a whole new level. This book is an absolute must read for anyone interested in making truly conscious food choices, and amazingly delicious Vegiterranean food!"

—BRENDA DAVIS RD, coauthor of
Becoming Vegan: Comprehensive and Express Editions

"*The Vegiterranean Diet* is wise, clear, complete, practical, and it celebrates real food that is really delicious. Julieanna Hever is adept at translating science into understandable terms, and with a great deal of heart, she's brought my Italian heritage and my vegan proclivities into perfect alignment."

—VICTORIA MORAN, author of *Main Street Vegan*
and director, Main Street Vegan Academy

"Julieanna Hever has knocked it out of the park with this grand slam of a book, as much a lifestyle plan as a diet alone. The first half is the most comprehensive review of why the Mediterranean basin is so attractive and associated with superior health. If every medical student read this, the health of the Western world would leap ahead in a few weeks. The recipes and kitchen skills are thorough and I cannot wait to try them."

—JOEL KAHN MD, FACC, Clinical Professor of Medicine, Wayne
State University SOM, author of *The Whole Heart Solution*

"In *The Vegiterranean Diet*, Julieanna Hever revolutionizes the Mediterranean diet with plant-based prowess. Backed by research, Julieanna's program serves up expert advice, meal plans, and irresistible, authentic recipes. Yet it's her unparalleled passion that truly inspires, through every page. Let Julieanna guide you to abundant health…the Vegiterranean way!"

—DREENA BURTON, author of *Plant-Powered Families*
and host of plantpoweredkitchen.com

"*The Vegiterranean Diet* is an inspiring example of 'take the best and leave the rest.' Grounded in the beauty of tradition, Julieanna Hever offers a delicious, whole-food version of Mediterranean cuisine and nutrition."

—MICAELA KARLSEN, MSPH,
Founder of PlantBasedResearch.org

"*The Vegiterranean Diet* is an approachable, yet science-based, read that further elevates our understanding of the Mediterranean Diet and the importance of whole-food, plant-based eating."

—ANDY BELLATTI, MS, RD,
Strategic Director, Dietitians For Professional Integrity

THE Vegiterranean DIET

The New and Improved
Mediterranean Eating Plan—
with Deliciously Satisfying
Vegan Recipes for Optimal Health

Julieanna Hever
MS, RD, CPT

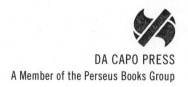

DA CAPO PRESS
A Member of the Perseus Books Group

Copyright © 2014 by Julieanna Hever

Printed in the United States of America.

For information, address Da Capo Press, 44 Farnsworth Street, 3rd Floor, Boston, MA 02210.

Set in 11.25 point Adobe Caslon Pro by Marcovaldo Productions, Inc., for the Perseus Books Group

Cataloging-in-Publication data for this book is available from the Library of Congress.
First Da Capo Press edition 2014
ISBN: 978-0-7382-1789-5 (paperback)
ISBN: 978-0-7382-1790-1 (e-book)

Published by Da Capo Press
A Member of the Perseus Books Group
www.dacapopress.com

Da Capo Press books are available at special discounts for bulk purchases in the U.S. by corporations, institutions, and other organizations. For more information, please contact the Special Markets Department at the Perseus Books Group, 2300 Chestnut Street, Suite 200, Philadelphia, PA, 19103, or call (800) 810-4145, ext. 5000, or e-mail special.markets@perseusbooks.com.

10 9 8 7 6 5 4 3 2 1

Contents

FOREWORD BY DR. NEAL BARNARD   vii
INTRODUZIONE   ix
HOW TO USE THIS BOOK   xiii

Parte Uno The Traditional Mediterranean Diet

1   The Birth of the Mediterranean Diet   3

2   The Benefits and Myths of the Mediterranean Diet   15

Parte Due The New and Improved Mediterranean Diet

3   The Three C's of How We Eat: Compassion,
    Carnism, and (Over)Consumption   41

4   The Veg Ten: Basics of the Vegiterranean Diet   61

Parte Tre Vegiterranean Every Day

5   The Vegiterranean Food Pyramid and Plate   89

6   Nutrizione: Essential Building Blocks
    of the Vegiterranean   109

7   *Stile de Vita:* Strategies, Meal Plans, and
    Navigating the World   143

8   *Un Giorno nella Vita:* The Vegiterranean Kitchen   167

9   *Buon Appetito!* The Recipes   181

RESOURCES 241

NUTRIENTS CHARTS AND TABLES 243

METRIC CONVERSION CHART 250

ACKNOWLEDGMENTS 251

ABOUT THE AUTHOR 253

NOTES 255

INDEX 263

Foreword

The Mediterranean Diet is on everyone's mind these days. More people than ever are looking to the coasts of France, Italy, Greece, and Lebanon, not just for romantic images of these beautiful lands, but for the delicious tastes and good health that come from their culinary traditions. And they are right. From the aromas of the kitchen and the flavors on the dinner table come an abundance of good health. Mediterranean diets are good for you.

But that M-word means different things to different people. For some it means a glass of wine. For someone else, it means olive oil. For others, it might mean favoring fish over beef. But what actually gets the credit for the healthfulness of the diets of Mediterranean countries? In 2009, a team of researchers tackled exactly that question. In the European Prospective Investigation into Cancer and Nutrition (EPIC) study, the research team examined 23,349 men and women living in Greece and tracked their health over an 8-year period. It turned out that the factors associated with health and longevity were: boosting vegetables, fruits, and nuts; avoiding meat; keeping alcohol intake moderate; minimizing animal fats in comparison with olive oil; and—perhaps surprisingly—avoiding fish and shellfish.

So what really gets the credit for health in the Mediterranean region is the prominence of fruits, vegetables, legumes, and grains and a general avoidance of the meaty diets that are commonplace in North America and much of the rest of the world. The people who take pride in their vegetables, fruits, and artisanal breads are those who are healthiest and live longest.

Years ago, a restaurateur in the south of France showed me how he selects fresh vegetables. Although we were talking about simple, everyday foods, he examined each one the way a jeweler would inspect a fine diamond. He had a deep understanding of the different varieties and carefully judged their quality and ripeness. While many in the U.S. think of green beans or asparagus as something that plops out of a can onto a side of the plate, he viewed them as nature's crowning achievements with enormous power for health.

That power is real. In our research studies at the Physicians Committee we have seen countless people use the power of nutrition to regain their health. People struggling with weight problems, diabetes, and chronic pain who adopt plant-based diets can revolutionize their health and feel better than they have in years.

The Vegiterranean Diet brings you the best of the Mediterranean. It takes full advantage of healthy traditions and brings it all to you in a simple, practical, and step-by-step method.

Neal D. Barnard, MD
Adjunct Associate Professor of Medicine
George Washington University School of Medicine
President, Physicians Committee for Responsible Medicine
Washington, DC

Introduzione

With an open heart, full mind, and complete candor, I'm ecstatic about sharing *The Vegiterranean Diet* with you. First and foremost, I wrote this book to put diet and health into both historical and global context, as well as to help shift our thinking so we can create a truly sustainable future. Several events inspired me to write this book. First, full disclosure: I am madly passionate about all things Mediterranean...especially Italian. After studying Renaissance art history and years of ancient Greek and Roman drama and literature from childhood through undergrad, my parents rewarded my sister and me when we graduated university by taking us to Italy. As soon as we set foot on *terra Italiano*, I was enamored. The food, the people, the history, the culture, (did I mention the food?), the architecture, the art, the fashion, the language...*che bella*! So deep is my amore for Italy, after playing Shakespeare's Juliet in a ninety-nine-seat theatre company I was a performer in (my fantasy-come-true), and having even named my two beloved dogs based on Italian coffee drinks (first Latte, now Cappuccino), I truly consider myself an Italian at heart.

Secondly, I fell in love with and married a man from the Mediterranean. He is responsible for connecting me to his mom, Miri—the talent who seeded my passion for Mediterranean cooking. Not many girls fall in love with their mothers-in-law so I feel blessed indeed. She makes gourmet, healthful cooking look easy and taste extraordinary. With no negative underpinnings, my mother-in-law is like a mad, brilliant scientist in the kitchen. Give her the ingredients and watch the magic unfold. In fact, working on recipes for this book was perhaps the most inspiring, exhilarating, and rewarding experience of my culinary career thus far.

Creating meals together in the kitchen with her genius and my crazy healthy demands enabled what I truly am proud to present here. Taking the oil out of a Mediterranean diet while keeping the flavor!? "Humph! Impossible," I was warned...but this is not so when your secret weapon is my mom-in-law!

Finally, I had the tough assignment to give a nutrition seminar in May 2013 on board a cruise in the Mediterranean. I know ... twist my rubber arm! It was there, in my stateroom on the ship, staring out into the deep blue sea, that this book was outlined and constructed. Traveling with my always adventurous and fun mom, we explored the Med from a vegan perspective, asking tour guides, restaurant owners, and waitstaff for plant-friendly options. Met with nothing but pure enthusiasm, we were guided through delectable, enchanting, and healthy experiences around Greece, Turkey, and Italy. Sitting on patios, by marinas, and in tiny cafes, we indulged in dolmas, broad beans, wild greens, eggplant salad, hummus, tahini, stews, fresh breads, salads, olives, vegetables, wines, and more. Traditional Mediterranean foods have it all. Satisfying and bursting with flavor, these foods also bestow ideal nutrition. It is no wonder the research has supported it as a gold standard for eating healthfully.

But what I recognized is that this is not unique to one region of the world. Instead, Mediterranean foods are the epitome of traditionalism, speaking the universal language of health! Around the globe, cultures have always eaten primarily whole plant foods, and the populations that remain successful with regard to their health are the ones that stick to their tradition. As a whole food herbivore traveling in the Med, my plant-goggles enabled me to see what we have lost in translation. As my mother-in-law demonstrates to me every time we cook together, whole plants are the staples, the crux of a health-promoting diet.

Processed and animal foods eaten in consistent doses were never the dietary norm, and this is how we ended up in our current healthcare crisis. Classically, a Mediterranean diet does include a small amount of animal products. However, as you will see in this book, we have come to a period of time where we can no longer partake in the extravagant usage of animals for food, as we have in the past few decades. It is without doubt wreaking havoc on our bodies and the Earth's resources and is causing tremendous suffering for humans and animals alike. We do not need animal products to survive, and we will thrive by switching to a whole food, plant-based lifestyle. It is time to go back to our roots, to enjoy the magnificence of modern healthcare *only* when needed, and to use diet and lifestyle as everyday medicine.

The flavors and foods of the Med, though incredibly delicious, are not exclusive, per se. Instead, it is the wholesome food groups they symbolize that is the secret of their success. Numerous cultures and countries border the Mediterranean, all with distinctive subtleties, yet with powerful health benefits. You will notice my *Italiano* bias throughout, just in language and play, but that is simply due to my love of Italy and as a representation of *all* the regions in that exquisite part of the world. The Mediterranean region revealed to us the secret of long-term health and disease prevention, and I will show you how and why these successful behaviors can easily be implemented into your life. This book is *me*—my heart, soul, mind, and passion—on a plate along with salad, hummus, and a glass of wine ... may it inspire you to eat and enjoy whole, plant foods ... TO YOUR HEALTH!

How to Use This Book

Like the variations in culture around the Mediterranean countries, this book peppers different personalities throughout the nine chapters. Front-loaded with the history and science, you should feel armed with the data as to why the Mediterranean diet is so successful and—perhaps, more importantly—why certain conclusions are off-base by the end of Parte Uno. In fact, if you are eager to jump into the juicy particulars of the lifestyle, feel free to skip the first two chapters—just promise you'll return!—to get the detailed scoop. Then, in Parte Due you will witness the passion behind my Vegiterranean thinking and explore the fundamental principles on how to eat this most health-promoting diet, from a nutrient standpoint and beyond. Next, Parte Tre illustrates the nuts and bolts of implementing Vegiterranean living in the real world, with strategies for behavior change, meal plans, and a whole lot more. Also in this section, you will be introduced to the Vegiterranean Kitchen, providing you with pages of tips for stocking your kitchen, subbing out ingredients for Vegi-friendly options, and loading up on delicious Vegiterranean recipes to enjoy on a day-to-day basis and impress your loved ones with. Ultimately, my goal is to broaden your skyline, offer a deliciously nutritious plan, and share the ethereal, awe-inspiring wholesomeness of the Vegiterranean way of life.

The Traditional Mediterranean Diet

CHAPTER 1

The Birth of the
Mediterranean Diet

As I sat in my stateroom, aboard the ship, throughout our brief, yet breathtaking exploration of the Mediterranean, I was mesmerized by the tranquility, the beauty, and—perhaps, mostly—the history. How extraordinary to be riding in the waters and flirting with the boundaries of multiple countries where Western civilization was birthed. Perhaps you have heard of the Mediterranean diet, or maybe even incorporated some of its deliciousness into your eating pattern. I am eager to share how it came to be revered and widely accepted as such a fabulous and health-promoting lifestyle. Although the history is long and extensive, the highlights and punctuations outlined in this chapter provide a necessary background to the Vegiterranean way.

History Points the Way to the Med Diet

Envision deep sapphire, calm waters, edges of islands boasting lush landscapes and undeniable antiquity, people rich with culture, and signature flavors. These previews only hint at the exquisiteness of the region known as the Mediterranean, which literally translates to "sea between lands." Bordered by three continents (Southern Europe, Western Asia, and Northern Africa) and at least eighteen nations—each unique in politics, religion, and ethnicity—the Mediterranean Sea is considered the incubator for

In this chapter, you'll learn...
- *The history of the traditional Mediterranean diet.*
- *What exactly the traditional Mediterranean diet is made of.*
- *How the Mediterranean diet protects against overall mortality and incidence of most major chronic degenerative diseases.*

Western civilization. Deeply rooted populations originating in the lands circling the Mediterranean Sea include those that shaped modern Western culture, like the Mesopotamians, Egyptians, Canaanites, Byzantines, Ottomans, Greeks, and Romans. This region is also the birthplace of the Hebrew, Islamic, and Christian religions. More recently, shortly after World War II, the peoples of this area inspired scientists to study the significant impact of diet and lifestyle on health. In the 1950s, the modern interpretation of the Mediterranean diet was born and grew to become known as the gold standard for a healthy eating pattern.

Long before current times, the healing properties of food were a part of the Med culture. In fifth century BC, the father of modern medicine, Hippocrates, famously decreed, "Let thy food be thy medicine, thy medicine be thy food," and dedicated his essay *On Diet* to nutrition and the role of diet as disease therapy; he also wrote *Corpus Hippocraticum*, an entire work centered on the importance of nutritional choices.

As one of the most renowned philosophers from Greek antiquity, Plato was well acquainted with multiple peoples from around the Mediterranean region. Plato's legendary teachings provide insight into the foods, customs, and dietary principles of his time. These references are mentioned consistently throughout his works, offering a peek into their significance in ancient Western culture. Plato is quoted in *Laws*, "For there ought to be no other secondary task to hinder the work of supplying the body with its proper exercise and nourishment." Plato preached moderation and self-restraint, repeatedly warning that excessive food intake and debauchery are unhealthy and lead to disease. In light of our focus here on a Vegiterranean Diet, we should take special note that Plato urged a plant-based diet, associating meat with obesity and illness, possibly attributable to his belief in soul reincarnation. Still, his main message was moderation and a balanced consumption of all kinds of nutrients in an effort to avoid dietary excesses and degenerative disease—a message we'd do well to heed in this day and age!

Fast Forward…Twentieth Century Disease Twist

Cardiovascular disease (CVD) is currently the world's number one killer. But it was not always this way. Communicable (a.k.a. infectious) diseases, accidents, and violence used to prevail as leading causes of death up until the mid-twentieth century when chronic disease took over. An increase in lifespan and decrease in mortality from communicable diseases occurred because of the discovery of antibiotics, use of childhood vaccinations, and advances in medical care, hygiene, and sanitation. In 1900, the leading causes of death were pneumonia, tuberculosis, diarrhea/enteritis, and diphtheria, which contributed to one-third of all deaths. In 1997, heart disease and cancers accounted for 54.7 percent of deaths, with only 4.5 percent attributable to communicable diseases. Trying to get to the bottom of this dramatic shift led to a fascinating onset of exploration by pioneering scientists and healthcare practitioners.

The bulk of health and nutrition investigation is concentrated on CVD for a couple of key reasons. As mentioned above, it is the number one cause of (mostly preventable) death around the world, in both developed and developing countries. Secondly, CVD incidence commonly occurs in populations with other chronic causes of death like cancers, diabetes, kidney disease, and Alzheimer's disease.

A new era in CVD research began in 1948: This was the year that the World Health Organization and the U.S. National Heart Institute (one of the first institutes of the National Institutes of Health, now called the National Heart, Lung, and Blood Institute) were founded, and the year that the American Heart Association reorganized into a public agency with a broader scope. Between 1948 and 1972, dozens of studies were performed around the world assessing CVD incidence and possible risk factors. These studies inspired early clinical trials with the overall goal of prevention. Ultimately, from these lessons learned, the "Mediterranean diet" as we know it now was born…

What Exactly Is the Traditional Mediterranean Diet?

Because of the vastness of locations and populations living on and near the Mediterranean Sea, there are variations of the Med Diet. Researchers agree that the traditional Mediterranean diet consists of:[1]

- Abundant plant foods: vegetables, fruits, cereals (including bread), legumes, nuts, and seeds;
- Minimally processed, seasonally fresh, locally grown foods;
- Olive oil as the primary source of fat;
- Fresh fruits for dessert on typical days;
- Dairy products in moderate amounts (mostly as cheese and yogurt);
- Zero to four eggs per week;
- Low consumption of meat and meat products;
- High monounsaturated to saturated fat ratio; and
- Moderate alcohol consumption, preferably from wine.

Essentially, this eating pattern is linked to the olive-cultivating regions of the Mediterranean (mostly Greece and Southern Italy) in the mid-twentieth century. Plant foods are the core while animal products are marginal. The practice of enjoying carefully prepared meals that are lengthy and relaxed is paired with lifestyle habits of regular physical activity, ample social support, and a sense of community. As a modern day dietitian writing from the center of a hugely urban, frenetic setting, this lifestyle feels peaceful, luxurious, and romantic—and one that might seem hard to attain. The good news is that a Med diet—and lifestyle—is achievable.

It All Began in Crete

Crete—the mountainous, elongated, most populated, and fifth-largest island in all of the Mediterranean—has an extensive and intriguing history but its relationship to the Mediterranean diet and all the research around it also begins in 1948. After World War II, Crete was ravaged and weak, torn by instability and lacking a solid economic and social structure to help its people thrive. A private organization from the United States, the Rockefeller Foundation, collaborated with the Greek government to attempt to improve the situation by diagnosing Crete's problems and helping to strategize solutions.[2] Led by epidemiologist Leland Allbaugh, a team assessed the current living standards on the island and made recommendations as to how to proceed proactively to improve conditions and maximize success of the island.

At the time, this survey was considered the best-known portrait of the food habits and nutrient intake in the Mediterranean basin. Researchers collected detailed data from 765 households to estimate annual food consumption, production, and purchase. According to this census, not much had changed in terms of diet in the many centuries between ancient Greece and 1948.

The Cretan diet consisted chiefly of foods of vegetable origin, with cereals, vegetables, fruits, and olive oil predominating. Pulses and nuts were eaten in appreciable quantities—especially during the winter—and potatoes were used quite extensively. On the other hand, meat, fish, milk, eggs, and sweets were consumed in relatively small amounts. Butter was seldom used.[3]

Typical Cretan folks spread their food intake evenly throughout the day, with approximately six light meals, always including bread and tea, coffee, or wine. Olives and olive oil provided the main source of fat, contributing heavily to total energy intake … so much so that "food seemed literally to be 'swimming' in oil."[4] Dessert was typically fresh, seasonal fruit, and sweets were not commonly served. Essentially, Cretans were the modern "farm to table" eaters, with diets based on locally grown and sourced foods.

A comparison of foods available in Crete and the US showed that 61 percent of total caloric intake was comprised of whole plant foods for the Cretans. (That number is larger when you include the fact that 78 percent of table fats were derived from olives and their oils.) Only 7 percent of calories in the Cretan diet came from animal products. Interestingly, the percentage of total calories from fat (including all sources) was approximately 38 percent, a number similar to that of the United States' diet during the same period; of course, this percentage is still higher than that recommended for chronic disease prevention today. Examinations coupled with feedback from local physicians showed that vitamin deficiency was not a significant issue. Thus, overall, the Cretan diet was found to be nutritionally adequate when compared to the United States National Research Council Recommended Dietary Allowances.

In 1948, Crete, along with Palestine and Cyprus, had the lowest mortality rates in the Mediterranean basin. Although overall mortality rates were similar between the United States and Crete, the causes of death were the polar opposite. Compared to the United States, Crete had four times as many deaths due to infectious disease per 100,000 people and 40 percent more tuberculosis, violent, and accidental deaths. However, death rates from cardiovascular disease, cancer, and kidney disease were one-third to one-fourth less in Crete, and cerebral hemorrhages were approximately one-half the number of those in the United States. In other words, Crete was experiencing a very low incidence of the chronic diseases that were three to four times more common in the United States, where meat, dairy, and sugar consumption was at least five times higher and the intake of whole plant foods was dramatically lower. (No, correlation doesn't equal causation, but these trends are worth noting!)

Ancel Keys and the Seven Countries Study

Dr. Ancel Keys, a man who accomplished quite an enormous and impressive list of contributions to human health in his 100 years of life, is the person responsible for the Mediterranean diet as we think of it today. An American physiologist, Keys founded the field known as quantitative human biology, invented the K ration (meals for troops in combat), wrote the most comprehensive account of the physiological, psychological, and cognitive effects of starvation (published as The Biology of Human Starvation, 1950), and is credited with connecting diet and cholesterol to cardiovascular disease risk.[5] In fact, his nickname was Mr. Cholesterol once his lipid hypothesis became widely accepted. Keys served as the chairman of the International Society of Cardiology, consulted with the World Health Organization and Food and Agricultural Organization, and was professor emeritus in the School of Public Health and former director of the University of Minnesota's Laboratory of Physiological Hygiene. Keys had a profound influence on physiology and health when he put saturated fat on the radar as a major factor in heart disease and was a pioneering champion for a low-fat diet and healthy lifestyle.

Keys began his years-long, international investigation on the connection between diet and cardiovascular disease after World War II. He was one of those open-minded, inquisitive scientists who recognized the aforementioned new trends emerging: those statistics from northern Europe indicating that mortality rate from coronary heart disease dropped significantly as food supplies became short; occurring around the same time as the epidemic of heart attacks suffered by American executives grew. He had also just finished his classic study on human semi-starvation, where he had illuminated the quick ability of the human body to rapidly change what were considered static characteristics, like morphology, physiology, biochemistry, and psychology. All of these factors encouraged Keys to dig deeper into discovering characteristics that may be related to the tendency to develop CVD.

One of the first formal studies of this period was the Minnesota Business and Professional Men's Study[6] led by Keys, Henry Taylor, and their colleagues. In it, they examined 281 "healthy" Minnesota business and professional men during a 15-year period, beginning in 1947, aiming to identify possible risk factors for heart disease. After measuring weight, body fatness, blood pressure, and blood cholesterol levels, they found that the only statistically significant predictor of future heart disease was a high total cholesterol level. Although this early study was too limited to produce more predictive data, the methodology set a historical model for more formal studies on CVD. Further, it posed critical questions about lifestyle risk factors and set a foundation for the Seven Countries Study and other definitive international trials that led to a crucial wealth of knowledge and, ultimately, health recommendations. Around the same time, the Framingham and other studies around the United States and additional countries had established similar findings linking CVD to elevated blood pressure, serum cholesterol levels, and cigarette smoking.

Prior to this point in time, family history and genetics were understood to be the major predictors of disease risk. Yet, Keys (and others) suspected there was more to this principle. In order to explore this further, Keys compared atherosclerosis and coronary heart disease incidence in middle-aged Japanese men living in their native country, Japan, to those living in Hawaii and in Los Angeles in 1956.[7] Because these men came from similar genetic backgrounds, it made for a good, built-in control system, enabling an evaluation of other possible non-genetic factors.

Keys found that coronary heart disease was very rare in Japan, but the Japanese living in the United States suffered the same high frequency of disease as the "local caucasians" and had similar cholesterol levels. Although their genetics had not changed when migrating to the United States, they acclimated their diet and lifestyle, thereby adopting the same incidence of coronary heart disease. The Japanese living in Los Angeles ate a diet with approximately 39 percent of their calories coming from fat compared to those in Japan who consumed somewhere between 9 to 14 percent. Keys concluded that although dietary fat cannot be the sole responsible factor for heart disease, the evidence was mounting in that direction.

Other researchers discovered similar results when comparing Japanese men in Japan, Hawaii, and California. (Note that similar findings were discovered later in one of the most comprehensive epidemiological studies of all time, the China Project, which occurred throughout the 1980s.[8] Studying 367 variables in 6,500 adults with similar genetics in 65 different counties in China, Dr. T. Colin Campbell, professor of nutritional biochemistry at Cornell University, and his colleagues found 8,000 statistically significant correlations between various dietary factors and disease. It was increasingly clear that although "genetics loads the gun, environment pulls the trigger."[9])

Building on all of this research, Keys and his colleagues began in 1957 what would eventually culminate in the landmark Seven Countries Study,[10] the first study to methodically evaluate the impact of diet and lifestyle on CVD risk in different populations throughout the world. Sixteen cohorts were selected from seven countries: Finland, Greece, Italy, Japan, The Netherlands, United States, and Yugoslavia. Approximately 13,000 working men, aged forty to fifty-nine, were examined and followed for approximately thirty years. Information on diet was randomly sampled and nutrient intake calculated for each cohort. Major differences were found in habitual dietary patterns as well as strongly contrasting CVD incidence between populations with the lowest rates found in Japan and the Greek islands and the highest in the United States and Finland (the twenty-five-year coronary heart disease mortality was highest in East Finland and lowest in Crete with a six-fold difference between these two populations). Overall, the Seven Countries Study provided compelling evidence that a diet consisting of less than 10 percent of calories from saturated fats and its associated lower serum cholesterol levels is necessary for a lower risk of CVD.[11]

Keys, along with his wife Margaret, went on to write the tome *Eat*

Well and Stay Well,[12] which summarized their best advice for preventing CVD, as well as providing some interesting insights to the philosophies, language, and nuances of the mid-twentieth century:

1. If you are fat, reduce.
2. Restrict use of fats in dairy products and in ordinary meats.
3. Use vegetable oils in cookery, not as medicine.
4. Avoid hydrogenated products but if you insist on a spread, use the newer margarines.
5. Avoid heavy use of salt and sugar.
6. Favor fish, shellfish, poultry, fresh vegetables, fruits, non-fat milk products.
7. Do not depend on the drugstore or vitamin peddlers for a good diet.
8. Be sensible about cigarettes, alcohol, excitement, business strain.
9. Get plenty of exercise, with recreation and work out-of-doors.
10. Learn more about cookery and have fun without saturation.

As pointed out by Dr. Marion Nestle,[13] nutrition, food studies, and public health professor at New York University, the Keys' recommendations look very similar to the Dietary Guidelines for Americans, the first of which were published in 1980[14] and have not changed much at all to this day:

1. Eat a variety of foods.
2. Maintain ideal weight.
3. Avoid too much fat, saturated fat, and cholesterol.
4. Eat foods with adequate starch and fiber.
5. Avoid too much sugar.
6. Avoid too much sodium.
7. If you drink alcohol, do so in moderation.

Keys' work also served as part of the foundation for the Mediterranean diet pyramid,[15] developed in 1993 as a collaborative effort between Oldways Preservation & Exchange Trust and Harvard School of Public Health. The pyramid was created to describe a dietary pattern that is not only health-promoting, but also "attractive for its famous palatability." (You'll find this pyramid, with more details, on page 90.)

Ultimately, Keys' body of work, along with his colleagues' and successors' studies, set the stage for dietary and health recommendations to prevent and treat CVD and other chronic diseases.

What the Research Means to You

Scientific research is designed to be one of the most objective ways of analyzing what we see in the world and translating it into guidelines for making the safest, healthiest, and best choices. Because of the aim for clarity, accuracy, and overall truth, science is as technical and perfectionistic as possible. Personally, I want people who design airplanes and buildings to be as precise as humanly possible! However, with diet and health, it is more challenging to be exact and near impossible to live up to scientific standards. And so we do the best with the tools we have. Many in the scientific community do not support using evidence from epidemiological studies as a basis for recommendations. Instead, these studies are used as a way to formulate questions and generate further information via randomized controlled clinical trials—the gold standard of research methodology. The collected information then can be translated into usable data. However, it is important to remember that researching food and dietary patterns is not the same as studying pharmaceuticals. In drug trials, it is easy to randomize people, blind them and the investigators, define parameters, and test for clear outcomes and possible side effects over a relatively short period of time. The same holds true for an isolated nutrient when given in supplement form. But these studies do not contribute to our knowledge of nutrition and health on a real-life level.

Studying food intake and dietary patterns in a population is difficult and expensive to perform adequately in order to end up with clear, generalizable, relevant, and statistically significant outcomes. Humans, food, and dietary patterns are intricately more multifaceted than can be easily summarized. We are simply too complex to be oversimplified! An ideal dietary randomized controlled trial would encompass controlling and documenting every bite of every meal of a large group of subjects over a very long period of time, and then continuously testing their biomarkers for health, clinical signs of wellness, illness, and ultimately, mortality. Factors that make studying diet perplexing include: it costs a ton of money and resources; people don't always stick to the same food intake, especially if it is not the type they are comfortable with; fabulous food synergy (which I will excitedly elaborate on in Chapter 2); and the sheer complexity of the human body. In other words, definitive diet research is not an easy task and requires multiple perspectives.

Thus, public dietary recommendations have been made primarily on epidemiological studies.[16] Although these studies are powerful at identifying possible associations between dietary elements and health outcomes, detecting measurement of such effects may be difficult.[17] Intervention trials are indeed necessary to clarify cause and effect and to attempt to eliminate confounding (any extra variable which may influence the results). Ultimately, a combination of large observational epidemiologic studies, carefully designed randomized controlled trials, and basic science studies emphasizing food synergy instead of just isolated nutrients needs to be the focus of future research in order to truly create reliable and well-rounded public health dietary advice.[18]

The Med Holds Steady

Notwithstanding, the wealth of potential that came about from the work on nutrition and health of the latter half of the twentieth century stirred up quite a bit of further clinical study. As expected, data vis-à-vis the so-called Mediterranean diet stood up to the more controlled testing and continues to impress researchers to this day. Two of the first major controlled trials on the Mediterranean diet are the Lyon Diet Heart Study and the PREDIMED trial (*Prevencion con Dieta Mediterranea*).

The Lyon Diet Heart Study[19] was the first trial to report health benefits from a "modernized" version of the Mediterranean diet.[20] It tested whether a Mediterranean dietary pattern would be more effective at preventing a recurrence of heart attack in those who had already experienced one, when compared to a standard recommended "heart-healthy" diet. Thus, this study focused on secondary prevention, looking to confirm a protective benefit for those who already had diagnosed CVD. The experimental group ate a Mediterranean-style diet comprised of an abundant consumption of fruits and vegetables, a low intake of meat and dairy, and the use of rapeseed oil, an oil rich in omega-3 alpha-linolenic acid (ALA) for nearly four years.

Despite similar risk factor profiles between the experimental and control groups, the people following the Mediterranean diet had a 50 percent decrease in risk of recurrent heart attack or CVD complications, as well as fewer cancers and a significant reduction in all-cause mortality.

Later, the PREDIMED[21] trial went out to seek similar results but in a primary prevention situation, where the population was at high risk for—but had not yet been diagnosed with—CVD. Three diets were compared: a Mediterranean diet supplemented with extra-virgin olive oil (EVOO), a Mediterranean diet supplemented with mixed nuts, and a control diet (where subjects were advised to reduce dietary fat—although intake ended up to be very high, it was still lower than the other two diets). No matter which diet, participants could eat however much they wanted. Ultimately, PREDIMED found a 30 percent relative stroke risk reduction in the group that supplemented with EVOO and a 46 percent reduction in risk in the nuts group when compared to the group eating the control diet.

Studies are ongoing, exploring all the possible reasons why the Mediterranean diet is so successful. As of now, research—which continues to pour in—shows that a Mediterranean diet provides significant protection against overall mortality and major chronic degenerative disease.[23] It is associated with fewer cardiovascular- and cancer-related deaths;[24] decreased risk of stroke and depression;[25] improved physical functioning, slower cognitive decline, and lower risk of developing Alzheimer's disease;[26] reduced prevalence of metabolic syndrome,[27] type 2 diabetes, and likely peripheral artery disease;[28] and better quality of life with aging.[29] Nutritional components of the Med diet have been found to have anti-inflammatory, anti-oxidative effects—which also have been shown to help prevent many chronic diseases.

CHAPTER 2

The Benefits and Myths of
the Mediterranean Diet

The Mediterranean diet is perhaps the most well studied diet of all time. And the momentum is not slowing down, either. This diet has unquestionably withstood the scrutiny and prevails as the gold standard in the diet world. What researchers have been trying to get to the bottom of in recent years is exactly *why* it works. In this chapter, I will dissect the details and describe precisely what makes the Med plan so powerful. On the flip side, I will also debunk the three most pervasive myths surrounding it. All of this info will prep you for the new, improved and even healthier Med diet ... the Vegiterranean way.

Five Reasons the Mediterranean Diet Works

REASON #1: THE MEDITERRANEAN DIET IS (AND ALWAYS HAS BEEN) A WHOLE FOOD, PLANT-BASED DIET

In this chapter you'll learn...
- *The top five reasons the Mediterranean diet is so effective, including the fact that it is—and always has been—a whole food, plant-based diet.*
- *Three of the most popular myths about the Mediterranean diet, such as that olive oil, red wine, and/or fish are magic elixirs.*
- *Olive oil is not the cornerstone to the traditional Med Diet's success.*
- *Opting for whole food sources of healthy fats is ideal in order to save hundreds of calories a day, increase fiber and nutrient intake, and manage essential fatty acid metabolism.*
- *Why fish is a less than ideal source of essential fats—and how to get omega-3 fats from plant foods.*

Planting Seeds

Although the term "plant-based" has risen in popularity in recent years, it is by no means a new way of eating. Diets were inherently plant-based since recorded history. In modern society, as our diets went awry and animal products moved toward the center of the plate, we needed to coin this new description, "plant-based," in order to shift back toward a more traditional, health-promoting way of eating. Anthropologists suggest that plant foods served as the primary source of energy in our ancestral lineage.[1] Carbohydrates, found primarily in plant foods, are the preferred fuel source for the brain and for immediate and sustained energy, key needs for survival. Also, in the natural environment, plant foods are more consistent and abundant while animal foods are unpredictable and more difficult to obtain. In a recent discovery, plant remains were found in the teeth of early humans dating from approximately two million years ago.[2] Scientists believe their diet consisted mostly of tree leaves, fruits, wood, bark, grasses, and sedges. "One thing people don't realize is that humans are basically grass eaters. We eat grass in the form of the grains we use to make breads, noodles, cereals, and beer and we eat animals that eat grass" reports Dr. Benjamin H. Passey, a geochemist from Johns Hopkins University.[3] He and his colleagues are trying to figure out at what point in evolutionary history this "addiction to grass" began. This recent evidence confirms other reports that *Homo sapiens* relied on grass seeds (starchy plants) for energy starting at least 105,000 years ago[4] and that Neanderthals found in the Mediterranean region and northwestern Europe not only consumed a variety of plant foods—including date palms, legumes, and grass seed starches—but began cooking them to increase their digestibility.[5] It has also been found that during the Paleolithic period, various wild plant grains were processed, perhaps even into flours.[6]

In analyzing the survey of Crete and the information gathered from the Mediterranean basin countries of the *Seven Countries Study*, we learned that animal products were saved as celebratory foods for holidays, served in condiment-size portions when available, or offered more sizably in rare times of abundance. On the Mediterranean diet pyramid, which will be illustrated in Chapter 5, fish, poultry, and eggs are up in the "eat a few times a week" category, and red meat has its own "eat a few times a month" section at the very top. Overall, animal products added up to approximately 10 percent of total calories in Crete. A plant-based diet, indeed.

Beyond the Med, our ancestors throughout history have relied strongly on plant-based diets. Animal products were generally consumed in lesser quantities. Typically reserved for the wealthier segments of populations and/or for celebrations and festivities, meat was considered a luxury, set aside in times of scarcity, like during war or poor economic times. With advancing technologies in the mid-twentieth century such as refrigeration and railroads, meat consumption became more accessible. With economic support by the government like subsidies for farmers and food guide dietary recommendations in the United States, animal product consumption became increasingly more frequent and common, eventually ending up at the center of the plate. In 1909, total meat availability was approximately 56.3 kilograms (124 pounds) per year in the United States, decreasing to 44.6 kilograms (98 pounds) per year in 1935 and skyrocketing to 91.2 kilograms (201 pounds) per year in 2007, according to Dr. Neal Barnard's study on food trends.[7] In that same study, cheese rose from 1.7 kilograms (3.7 pounds) per year in 1909 to 14.9 kilograms (33 pounds) per year in 2007. These increases are dramatic. Animal foods were never eaten in the same abundance as they have been in these past several decades ... not even close. Our MAD (Modern American Diet), SAD (Standard American Diet) emphasis on eating farmed animals, their byproducts, and processed foods is what initiated the physical health, economic, environmental, public health, and animal welfare problems of today.

> **A plant-based diet technically means a diet that includes primarily or exclusively foods of plant origin. A vegan diet is one that is devoid of all animal products. A vegetarian diet typically refers to a lacto-ovo vegetarian pattern of eating, one that includes eggs and dairy, but eschews flesh.**
>
> VEGI-SIDE

Plant-Based for Overall Health

Although one can make the argument that an exclusively plant-based diet was not the norm throughout history, the research we have today endorses its extraordinary health benefits. At present, there is a substantial body of evidence showing that plant-based diets promote effortless weight management, increase longevity, and enhance protection against most chronic diseases. Plant-based diets are associated with lower overall and ischemic heart disease mortality,[8] decreased incidence of certain cancers,[9] lower overall blood pressure and incidence of hypertension, lower body weight and body mass index (BMI), more optimal cholesterol profiles, lower blood concentrations of C-reactive protein and other markers of inflammation, improved insulin sensitivity, and better glycemic control in people with diabetes.[10] The research is so persuasive that Kaiser Permanente, one of the leading HMOs in the United States, published a nutritional update[11] for physicians in their journal in spring of 2013 recommending physicians guide their patients toward eating a plant-based diet.

Plant-based diets are therapeutic in so many wonderful ways. To sum it up, it all comes down to the packaging. Comparing animal products to plant foods for nutrition is like comparing beige to a rainbow for color. Sure, animal products contain some nutrients that humans are adapted to use. But they also contain injurious components. Most importantly, humans do not need animal products to survive. In fact, we can easily do better without them. Nutrients found in animal products can be found better in plants.

What's Really in that Burger?

Some non-nutrient ingredients built into animal products—but not plants—include hormones such as insulin-like growth factor 1 (IGF-1). Consuming IGF-1 raises blood levels of the hormone. Further, the amino acid profile typical of animal protein increases our body's own production of IGF-1. As a full-grown adult, the goal is to slow down cell growth, not to accelerate it. Thus, IGF-1 promotes cancer growth.

Interestingly, a small population of individuals are born with an impaired ability to process growth hormone, like IGF-1.[12] This very rare condition, Laron syndrome, causes them to be short in stature, but they also enjoy the miracle of being free of cancer, type 2 diabetes, and acne. Research on this small group of people has reinforced the impact of a western diet on health, serving as a unique comparison.

Antibiotics are another bonus, non-nutrient feature of animal foods. An estimated 70 to 80 percent of antibiotics sold in the United States are used for factory-farmed animal production. Antibiotics are used in livestock production to promote rapid growth and to prevent infectious diseases, since the animals are bred and raised in unnaturally confined and stressful environments where illnesses spread quickly. We are at the pinnacle of imminent threat of antibiotic resistance, as people are dying of medication-resistant infections. Bacteria adapt and evolve very swiftly, and they are rapidly outsmarting researchers in the lab. As we create stronger antibiotics, the bacteria create stronger resistance to them. What does this mean for us? Previously preventable illnesses perpetuate. In 2013, the CDC estimated (conservatively, in their words) that more than two million people in America are needlessly sickened by antibiotic-resistant bacteria every year ... and that 23,000 die as a result. With our overuse of antibiotics—the vast majority due to animal food production—we are making many medications obsolete and facing superinfections as never before.

But wait, there's more: additional harmful toxins are unleashed when meats are cooked. A group of about 100 chemicals, collectively called polycyclic aromatic hydrocarbons (PAHs), are formed by the incomplete burning of organic substances such as wood, gas, coal, oil, and food. Smoking, grilling, broiling, or other high-heat methods of cooking meat lead to the development of PAHs. Raw foods, like fruits and vegetables, can also contain low levels of some PAHs because of environmental contamination in the soil and air. PAHs have been linked to increased cancer risk, and food is responsible for the majority of exposure. This is just the tip of the iceberg. Other compounds formed by high-temperature cooking of meat, poultry, fish, or eggs are heterocyclic amines (HCAs). HCAs are formed by the combination of creatine (a substance found in muscle), amino acids, and sugar over high heat. Higher temperatures and longer cooking times increase their development. Intakes

IGF-1 is naturally occurring in animal products, so it does not help to eat the organic or "hormone-free" versions.

VEGI-SIDE

of PAHs and HCAs may be associated with an increased risk of cancers,[13] especially stomach, colorectal, pancreatic, prostate, and breast. Yet another detrimental group of compounds formed by cooking meat includes advanced glycation end products (AGEs). Dietary AGEs contribute to oxidation and inflammation, which are central to the process of developing type 2 diabetes, cardiovascular disease, Alzheimer's, and most degenerative disease. AGEs are created through the Maillard, or nonenzymatic browning, reaction that occurs between sugars and free amino acids, lipids, or nucleic acids at high temperatures. These compounds are absorbed into the body, where they kick off catastrophic cascades. Highest levels of AGEs are found in beef, cheese, poultry, pork, fish, and eggs, and they are also found in hefty doses in butter, cream cheese, margarine, and mayonnaise.[14] Plant-based foods tend to have very few AGEs, even after cooking. Small amounts can be found in processed dry-heat foods, such as crackers, cookies, chips, etc., but probably because of the added high fat ingredients, like butter, and because of the protective factors in plants.

More recently, two additional compounds found in meat have been reported to produce negative health effects. One is *N*-glycolylneuraminic acid (Neu5Gc), which has been found to promote chronic inflammation, accelerating growth of tumor cells.[15] The other compound is trimethylamine *N*-oxide (TMAO). This made headlines recently when it was shown that meat eaters—but not herbivores—convert carnitine (an amino acid found primarily in meat) into TMAO via intestinal bacteria. High levels of TMAO have been associated with an increased risk for inflammation, atherosclerosis, heart attack, stroke, and death.[16]

But I Need Iron!

Easily absorbed iron is another reason people seek out animal products; ironically, heme iron—the type found in red meat, poultry, and seafood—adds harmful elements to the diet. Heme iron, touted for its better absorbability by most physicians, is the first-line recommendation to anemic patients as opposed to plant sourced nonheme iron. While heme iron is more completely absorbed, the body is less able to regulate it. Pro-oxidative and toxic to the cells, excess iron kicks off free radical formation. This translates to a possible link between heme iron intake and atherosclerosis, kidney damage, increased risk of heart attacks in men,[17] CVD in diabetic women,[18] and multiple types of cancers.[19]

Iron is stored in the body and is hard to get rid of. Although much of this research is somewhat conflicted and inconclusive, the possibility exists that high levels of iron may contribute to chronic disease.[20] Either way, eating animals for the iron is at best, unnecessary, and, at worst, harmful.

Nonheme iron is widely available from plants like leafy greens, beans, and oatmeal. Eating a healthy array of these foods and eating them together with a source of vitamin C (found in fruits and vegetables) that aids in absorption will prevent both iron deficiency and the pro-oxidative effects of excess iron.

Plant foods contain a massive surplus of health-promoting vitamins, minerals, fibers, and phytonutrients such as carotenoids, flavonoids, lignins, phytosterols, and phenolic acids, just to name a few. They truly are the world's most nutrient-dense, calorically light foods.

Whole Foods

Beyond the "plant-based" component of *whole food, plant-based*, "whole" is a whole other health proclamation. Eating food as food is becoming a lost art, thanks to brilliant science, engineering, and chemistry. Nowadays, all you have to do is look at a food label on most any packaged food product to see the transformation. Typically, processed foods contain unrecognizable, unpronounceable ingredients added for the purpose of preservation, nutrient enhancement, thickening, stabilizing, coloring, sweetening, and/or flavoring. Food in packages hardly resembles real food anymore—so much so that it is difficult to decipher what real food really is. Cooking is also dramatically different now. Instead of cooking over a stove with fresh, intact ingredients, we reheat in microwaves, use pre-prepared foods and convenience items more and more ... and that is only if we are eating at home in the first place. Half of our food dollars are spent eating outside the home.

Essentially, the marriage of today's described "whole food, plant-based" way of eating to the Mediterranean diet of the past—*a la* The Vegiterranean Diet—was intrinsic. We just need to repurpose it in the context of today by eliminating animal products, as well as processed foods which weren't even a part of the original plan!

REASON #2: SYNERGY

Synergy is defined as "the interaction or cooperation of two or more organizations, substances, or other agents to produce a combined effect greater than the sum of their separate effects."[21] In other words, one plus one equals three. For instance, take the human body and add food. The human body is magnificent in its intricacy. Consisting of approximately 100 trillion cells, 10 times that amount of microbial cells, 23 sets of chromosomes, 206 bones, 642 skeletal muscles, 11 organ systems, and a highly controversial, fluctuating estimated 22,333 genes,[22] our bodies are beyond brilliant. Biochemical and neurological reactions are occurring at an incalculable rate during every second of our lives. Science has made leaps and bounds when it comes to understanding anatomy and physiology— yet we have only just begun to tap into the infinite molecules of water in the true ocean of our complexity.

Consider, then, the anatomy of a whole, plant food. Take the humble tomato, for example. Literally hundreds of varieties are grown today, and likely tens of thousands of nutrients can be found in each variety. But one medium-sized raw red tomato, averaged for the annual and local fluctuations in nutrient content, contains: 22 calories, 1 gram protein, 0.25 gram fat, 4.78 grams carbohydrates, 1.5 grams fiber, 3.23 grams sugar, 12 milligrams calcium, 0.33 milligrams iron, 14 milligrams magnesium, 30 milligrams phosphorus, 292 milligrams potassium, 6 milligrams sodium, 0.21 milligrams zinc, 16.9 milligrams vitamin C, 18 micrograms folate, 1,025 international units vitamin A, 0.66 milligrams vitamin E, and 9.7 micrograms vitamin K. Tomatoes are super strong in the antioxidant department as they are loaded with carotenoids, flavonones, flavonols, hydroxycinnamic acids, glycosides, and more. The carotenoids found in tomatoes, being fat-soluble nutrients, are better absorbed when heated and consumed with a bit of fat. This is an example of food synergy. As defined in a stunningly articulated article explaining food synergy,[23] "Food in its natural form is a nonrandom mixture of numerous molecules, orchestrated evolutionarily to maintain the life of the organism being eaten."

Two Superlative Samples of Synergy:
The Beta-Carotene Trials and Sofrito

Beta-carotene is one of approximately 600 carotenoids found in plant foods, mostly red, orange, yellow, and green fruits and veggies, and it was the first of the bunch to become famous. Its antioxidant power was promising. Lung cancer, being one of the most common malignant tumors worldwide, is an area of important preventive research. In the 1980s, researchers noted that smokers with lung cancer tended not to eat adequate fruits and vegetables and that they consistently had low blood levels of beta-carotene. Therefore, researchers hypothesized that beta-carotene was protective against lung cancer and in early observational studies, beta-carotene appeared to have the potential to be a wonder drug to cure cancer. When push came to shove and researchers took to testing this theory in randomized controlled trials, the results were not exactly as anticipated.

One study,[24] the ATBC cancer prevention trial, divided up 29,133 male smokers from Finland into four groups: alpha-tocopherol (one form of vitamin E) supplements alone, beta-carotene alone, both alpha-tocopherol and beta-carotene, or placebo. Not only was no improvement found in the group given beta-carotene over the group provided the placebo, but the group taking the beta-carotene supplements had an 18 percent higher incidence of lung cancer than the placebo group! A couple of years later, another trial[25] was published (fittingly called the CARET study) where researchers gave 18,314 men and women who were at high risk of lung cancer either a combination of beta-carotene and vitamin A or a placebo. The intervention was stopped 21 months early due to substantial evidence of harm. In fact, the treatment group recorded 28 percent more lung cancer and 17 percent more deaths than the placebo group! Clearly, something was wrong with isolating and concentrating one carotenoid out of the hundreds, and it responded rather differently in the body than in theory. Still, when researchers went back[26] to the ATBC population and analyzed their baseline blood levels of carotenoids, they concluded that the consumption of several carotenoids from carotenoid-rich food sources is inversely related to lung cancer risk. This, by the way, was especially true with lycopene, as found in tomatoes and tomato products ... which brings us back to *sofrito*.

Sofrito is a sauce commonly used in Latin America and the Mediterranean region. A simple, yet popularly potent combination of tomato, onion, garlic, and olive oil, though the recipe fluctuates depending on which country you ask. Why is a marinara- or salsa-type sauce so special, you might wonder? Synergy. Gorgeous reactions occur with a combo food such as this. With heat over time, the tomato's carotenoids break down and combine with the fat of the oil and the phytochemicals of the garlic and onions. That is where the magic begins. The vitamin C in the tomato and the fat in the oil help the absorption of the carotenoids and other polyphenols found in this sauce. Studies actually show that the bioactivity of this sauce reacts synergistically to help prevent CVD and cancer. Seriously. And, this links back to the Mediterranean diet because this sauce is a staple there.

Clearly, the whole is greater than the sum of its parts. The isolated beta-carotene trials did not work because the other synergistic compounds were removed from beta-carotene-rich foods from which the benefit stems. Different bioactive nutrients work together and strengthen one another, enabling the greater good to manifest. Simply isolating one micronutrient (like beta-carotene) or one macronutrient (like protein) and expecting it to impart beneficial results defies the laws of physiology. This concept, known as reductionism, has been shown over and over again in research to fail. Eating a highly processed, refined food, sprayed with a multivitamin and claiming to meet the daily requirements of certain nutrients, for example, does not make it healthful. Nor does it make it a whole food ... and the body cannot be fooled. Similarly, fad weight-loss diets are predicated on the idea that you can vilify or evangelize a certain nutrient or food group. Eliminating carbohydrates, for example, is not only detrimental to your health, but research does not show this method of weight reduction to be preferable to a healthier option. The reason the Mediterranean diet works and has been shown to be consistently beneficial is because there is a combination of whole foods at its foundation, thereby supporting the principles of synergy.

REASON #3: IT IS AN OVERALL LIFESTYLE, NOT SIMPLY A DIET

Consider the dinner table. Not just any dinner table—*your* dinner table. How often do you sit down with a bottle of wine (or a pitcher of water), family, and/or friends, and enjoy a lovely, relaxing, extended meal—filled with whole-grain breads, soups, salads, fruits, grains, beans, classic masterpieces, and favorite traditional recipes with olives and nuts on the side as condiments; a meal seasoned with laughter and conversation, lively political debates, catching up on gossip, and updates of days gone by. Good food allows us opportunities to engage, connect, bond, and break bread together. For me, this conjures up feelings of comfort, celebration, and calm. And yet, this is not a daily, or even weekly, occurrence in most homes anymore (mine included). In many homes around the world, meals have devolved from mealtimes to food opportunities, from experience to requirement, and from nourishment to eating. In the Med and in the Blue Zone[27] societies, where longevity and health soar, eating is more of an experience, something that would be lovely to aspire to incorporate more into our busy lives, if and when possible. Food used to be created with care and intention. It was grown and nurtured. Dishes took time to prepare. Chemicals were not used to produce massive amounts of product. Processing meant chopping and cooking; nowadays, the term "natural" can legally appear on labels of foods processed with any of hundreds of additives. What's missing from our food is the food.

But beyond food, the Mediterranean success was so much more. The traditional people studied were very active, performing rigorous physical activity daily for work, lifting heavy equipment, farming, gardening, walking an average of five or so miles a day. According to the World Health Organization, physical inactivity is now the fourth leading risk factor for global mortality. Approximately 31 percent of adults around the world are insufficiently active. This statistic does not even refer simply to formal exercise ... just movement. We are not moving enough and that is crippling our bodies. Two of my favorite expressions from my personal-training days are: "Use it or lose it" and "You will rust out before you wear out." True indeed. The complex human body is designed to move; to stretch muscles; to make the heart pump blood throughout the circulatory system; to flex lymph through the lymphatic system, stimulating immune function; and to stress the bones and muscles to stimulate remodeling. Moving feels expected, easy, natural, and necessary. Sitting is crumpling, inhibiting, and wasteful. A crucial component to health, moving—and moving often—is the only way to thrive, continue activities of daily living, and sustain vitality.

In addition to food and physical activity, other lifestyle factors impact our health, including stress, smoking, and alcohol consumption. Stress is a harmful habit and a hallmark of our modern lifestyle. Being under the spell of daily stress promotes a constant hormonal cascade simulating the fight or flight response, repeatedly flooding our bodies with cortisol and adrenaline. Over time, this response impacts immune function, memory and cognition, mood, weight, digestion, and more. Although it is difficult to prevent stress in our lives, behaviors like exercise, mindfulness practice, and meditation can help our bodies handle and recover from those stressors. Smoking harms most organs in the body and is a known risk factor for disease—especially CVD and lung cancer. It is responsible for approximately 480,000 deaths a year in the United States alone, and the CDC estimates that 10 times more people have died prematurely from cigarettes than in all the wars fought in all of United States' history.[28] Alcohol is less black-and-white, as will be discussed later, but when consumed in moderation, as in the traditional Med diet, it can be safe and even beneficial. Yet in greater quantities, it is toxic—in-toxic-ating—and can cause problems.

It's All In Your Genes

Epigenetics[29] is the exploding field of study showing that lifestyle and diet determines whether or not your genes are switched on or lie dormant. "Epi-" is Greek for "around, over, after, above, and upon." Genetics is the study of heredity and the variety of inherited characteristics. Epigenetics looks at factors that may act around, over, after, above, and upon your DNA. The easiest way to understand how it works is to note that it takes multiple generations to see a true genetic adaptation from the environment show up in the gene pool. The fact that chronic diseases have increased in prevalence at speedy rates hints that it is not simply that more people have the genes for those diseases. Rather, it is environmental factors, especially diet, coming into play instead. Further, migrant studies (like the ones discussed in the previous chapter) are fascinating and informative, demonstrating people with similar genes having different health outcomes based on diet and lifestyle. Recent studies in epigenetics show promise of pinpointing mechanisms by which environment changes the outcome of genetic predisposition. That lifestyle can literally decide which genes are expressed and which remain dormant, and is rather empowering! We are not at the destiny of our genes; we are not victims. Instead, we can make choices to influence our health positively.

REASON #4: LESS IS MORE

There is a principle practiced in Japan (especially Okinawa) called *hara hachi bu*, which literally translates to "eat until you are 80 percent full." This common habit is perhaps one of the most powerful keys to eating that, in and of itself, could make a significant impact on your health. First, it dramatically adds mindfulness to your eating. Secondly, it prevents overeating. Overeating is silently ruining our health. Plato wrote of the harms of excessive intake, castigating it as an unhealthy habit way back in Greek antiquity.[30] Excess weight does not simply mean you may not fit into your skinny jeans. Instead, overweight and obesity are linked directly to multiple comorbidities like CVD, cancers, type 2 diabetes, osteoarthritis, aches and pains, sleep apnea, metabolic syndrome, gallbladder disease, fatty liver disease, infertility, pregnancy complications, and more.

Because we are faced with approximately 200 food choices a day and seductive, calorically dense options are available at all times of the day, overconsumption is now way too convenient. It takes approximately 3,500 calories to equal a pound so trimming off a few calories here and there makes a significant difference over time. A 20-percent reduction in intake, as in *hara hachi bu*, could lead to an effortless weight loss. In a hypothetical 2,500-calories-per-day diet, cutting 20 percent equals 500 calories per day, which is a one-pound a week weight loss. To make the calorie reduction less noticeable, you could simply take off 10 percent of calories from food intake and then make sure you are burning the other 10 percent of calories from daily exercise to end up with a similar result. Granted, calorie reduction is not as simple as it sounds on paper; there are many elements to it—which is why the whole concept of dieting is a mass failure. Building consistent habits, like aiming to eat until you are 80-percent satisfied, brings long-lasting results. Relying on rigid portion control, extreme restriction, and eating low satiety foods are recipes for disaster, as being hungry is not only uncomfortable but is also unsustainable because we are biologically designed to seek enough food to survive. Eating Vegiterranean, however, makes a dramatic difference. Vegiterraneans, like Okinawans, can naturally eat more food, but with fewer calories, thanks to the high quantity of fiber and water. Although thousands of diet books, pills, supplements, medications, and procedures promise easy weight loss, all roads eventually lead to calorie reduction. Therein lies the beauty of *hara hachi bu*. Even more beautiful are the principles of eating Vegiterranean—more food, fewer calories!

REASON #5: DELIZIOSA CUCINA!

How does a meal of warm Baked Oat Bread with Potato Corn Chowder, Falafel, White Bean and Rosemary dip, and Chocolate Hazelnut Chia Pudding for dessert sound? Or what about a Hearty Red Lentil Stew with Stone-Ground Cornbread and Grilled Nectarines with Amaretto Gelato to top it off? Vegiterranean dishes are classically delicious and satisfying—which helps you to stick to the plan (compliance is crucial for long-term benefit). The palatability and versatility of this type of cuisine is part of the charm, making sticking to it effortless.

Three Myths about the Traditional Mediterranean Diet

Now that we've tackled the reasons the Med is so effective, here are the most common misconceptions about the diet.

MYTH #1: OLIVE OIL IS A MAGIC ELIXIR

Oils and fats are perhaps the biggest sources of controversy in nutrition circles. How much fat is ideal as a percentage of total calories? Which types of fats and oils are preferable? To this day, the details are still slightly malleable and fluctuate as new research emerges. From a macroscopic perspective, a resounding dispute is whether a low-fat diet trumps a moderate-fat diet for weight management and disease prevention. On one side of the discussion is the low-fat camp, substantiated by the trailblazing research of Nathan Pritikin, Dr. Dean Ornish, and Dr. Caldwell Esselstyn— where they were able to reverse advanced CVD and rapidly and significantly reduce angina (chest pain) with a very-low-fat plant-based diet (about 10 percent of calories from fat) and lifestyle modification. Dr. Neal Barnard of the Physicians Committee for Responsible Medicine has shown dramatic improvement of type 2 diabetes with a similar diet.[31] Another critical piece in this puzzle is the fact that traditional rural Asian populations rank high in health with very low incidence of chronic disease compared to the rest of the world. In the Seven Countries Study, the Japanese (who derived approximately 10 to 15 percent of calories from fat) came in close after Crete in incidence of CVD. In The China Study,[32] Dr. Campbell and his colleagues determined that the rural Chinese dietary pattern in the 1980s, which averaged 14.5 percent calories from fat, espoused greater health benefits when compared to the more modernized regions of China. In fact, the death rate from CVD was 17 times higher in American men than in the men in rural China, and the American death rate from breast cancer was found to be five times higher than the rural Chinese at that time! Further, Okinawa, Japan, is one of the few regions in the world where the most centenarians (people age 100 and older) live and their incidence of chronic disease is significantly lower than that of the rest of the world. They traditionally eat a very-low-fat diet, as well.

The other side of this fascinating and ever-evolving deliberation is clearly and powerfully illustrated by the Mediterranean diet. As we saw in Crete, fat percentages were upwards of 35 to 40 percent of total calories, considered high when compared to the aforementioned low-fat diets. Yet, during the snapshot of this population, they had the longest life expectancy known at the time! Additionally, recent evidence supporting significant health benefits from consumption of high-fat foods, like nuts and seeds, begs further consideration for space in a healthy dietary pattern for more moderate levels of fat. The vegan population includes a small subset of people who maintain extensively raw diets, thereby tending to consume higher levels of fat. Nuts, seeds, and raw oils provide the bulk of their calories as they replace cooked staple foods like whole grains, starchy vegetables, and legumes, which are avoided. Although the research on raw foodists is not extensive, some studies have shown improved markers protective against cancer and CVD, as well as nutrient adequacy with the consumption of higher-fat, uncooked vegan diets.

Essentially, it is becoming evident that the *type* of fat is significantly more crucial to health, weight management, and longevity than the actual *amount* of fat, assuming calorie intake is balanced (a critical factor). In January 2014,[33] the Academy of Nutrition and Dietetics (AND, the leading organization for Registered Dietitians) revised its position on fatty acids for healthy adults, recommending an intake of 20 to 35 percent of total calories from fats with guidelines on the distribution of the types of fatty acids within that percentage. Specifically, it emphasizes consumption of omega-3 polyunsaturated fats (PUFAs) and advocates limiting saturated fats (SFAs) and trans fats (TFAs). The Institute of Medicine, American Heart Association, World Health Organization/ Food and Agricultural Organization, and European Food Safety Authority harmonize with this recommendation. Herein seems to be a happy compromise ... an olive branch, if you will.

VEGI-SIDE

Protagoras recommended that "all doctors forbid the sick to take oil, except the smallest quantity, if one is going to eat" because olive oil "is good for the outward parts of man's body [for anointing the skin], but at the same time as bad as can be for the inward."[34] Plato recommended that although olive oil "is helpful," it should not be a centerpiece of the diet.

So...What Are the Best Sources of Dietary Fat?

Is oil a healthy option? Many experts disagree on these specifics, too. Here is what we know about oils, in general:

All oils are pure, concentrated, 100 percent fat, containing approximately 120 calories and 14 grams of fat per tablespoon. Oils are processed and, therefore, stripped of all their fiber. They are significantly lower in micronutrients when compared to their whole food source, placing them at the bottom of the totem pole in terms of nutrient density. Further, oils are vulnerable to rancidity from cooking, aging, or improper storage. Some oils display this effect more than others, but this is something to consider as well. In order to illustrate the difference in quality between oil and its original source, let's anatomize the olive.

The nutritional anatomy of olives versus olive oil[35]

Nutrient	Olives (per 100 g)	Olive Oil (per 100 g)
Calories	115	884
Protein (g)	0.84	0
Total fat (g)	10.68	100.0
Carbohydrate (g)	6.26	0
Fiber (g)	3.20	0
Calcium (mg)	88	1
Iron (mg)	3.30	0.56
Magnesium (mg)	4	0
Phosphorus (mg)	3	0
Potassium (mg)	8	1
Sodium (mg)	735	2
Zinc (mg)	0.22	0
Vitamin A (IU)	403	0
Vitamin E (mg)	1.65	14.35

The nutritional difference between an olive and its expressed oil is quite pronounced, particularly when noting that the oil contains nearly eight times the amount of calories and more than nine times the grams of fat. The laws of nutrient density show that oil simply provides the lesser nutritional bang for your caloric buck. Allowing this comparison to be representative of most whole food sources of fats versus their extracted oils, the answer becomes clearer. Whole, intact sources of fat provide not only those healthy fatty acids but are higher in micronutrients and—perhaps more importantly—maintain their crucial fiber component. Consume the whole foods, and we enable synergy to do its job.

Olive Oil and the Fatty Acid Lowdown

What about olive oil, specifically? Let's deconstruct this further. Olive oil's primary fatty acid is monounsaturated. Broken down, it contains: 75 percent calories from MUFAs (primarily oleic acid), 14 percent calories from SFAs, and 11 percent calories from PUFAs. In nutrition science, individual macronutrients are studied in humans by comparing the same amount of calories coming from different macronutrients. For example, say hypothetically that the test group is given 300 calories of foods high in MUFAs and the control group is given those same 300 calories but from foods high in PUFAs. So the MUFA calories are being compared to the PUFA calories. The displacement or replacement of calories is what is being analyzed in these studies. Then, researchers can test statistically whether associations between those calories and hypothesized health outcomes exist (e.g., decreased blood pressure). So, back to our olive oil conundrum...

Recent evidence on fatty acids shows that MUFAs may have favorable effects on serum cholesterol. Decreased total- and LDL-cholesterol levels are found when MUFAs replace SFAs. When replacing carbohydrates, MUFAs seem to lower triglycerides and raise HDL-cholesterol. These are all health-promoting changes. Ah, but the plot thickens. When compared to PUFAs, MUFAs don't fare as well in some of the newest studies. More specifically, some data show that PUFAs decrease risk for CVD when replacing SFAs, but that MUFAs show a neutral effect. But, alas, the conclusions are inconclusive.

The good news is, as the 2014 AND Position Paper states, "these trials, coupled with observational, epidemiologic, and mechanistic studies, provide valuable evidence on the health effects of dietary fat and specific fatty acids." And as the clever and wise nutrition guru Dr. Michael Greger told me, "people don't eat MUFAs, PUFAs, or LOOFAHs." Ha! So true! What matters most is determining how this translates into the real world.

So you might be thinking, "Ok, if olive oil worked wonders in the traditional Mediterranean diet and appears to show benefits in more current research, isn't this the secret ingredient we need to incorporate into our diets?" Not so fast. This is a very loaded question and needs to be analyzed with a fine-toothed comb. Is it really the olive oil that is deserving of all the praise?

A whole food, plant-based diet in general—such as that of the traditional Mediterranean population—provides a colossal variety of phytochemicals, and olive oil is merely one possible source of many. Besides those befuddling fatty acids, olives and olive oil (especially extra-virgin olive oil) also contain a concentrated amount of phytochemicals that are exceedingly healthful and protect against oxidation and inflammation, understood to be potentially the fire flaming all illness. Just *some* of the myriad phytochemicals found in olives include (but are not limited to): phenols (hydroxytyrosol), terpenes (oleuropein), flavones (apigenin and luteolin), hydroxicinnamic acids (caffeic acid, cinnamic acid, ferulic acid, and coumaric acid), anthocyanidins, flavanols (quercetin and kaempferol), hydroxybenzoic acids, and hydroxyphenylacetic acids. Quite a bit of research suggests the beneficial impact of these compounds on protecting against CVD, cancers, osteoporosis, hypertension, and likely more. Thus, nutrients other than the fat content itself may very well deserve the credit for the health benefits of the diet. Additionally, the inclusion of olive oil in this diet encouraged the consumption of more vegetables, both cooked and as salads, since it is thought to enhance palatability. Of course, vegetables are extraordinarily packed with health-promoting nutrients! So it may not be the olive oil itself—but the whole foods ingredients accompanying it.

Perhaps the most unique consideration is that the context of how we live now has changed substantially in the past several decades. Calories are up against an entirely different framework. In post–World War II Crete and the Seven Countries Study, where food was not as accessible and abundant as it is today, olive oil helped substantiate total caloric intake for the people studied. This may be part of the reason they fared so well. And they were generally very active, walking miles each day and performing physically demanding work, thereby increasing their energy requirements. Because of the fact that now, in this second decade of the new millennium, at least one-third of the global population is overweight or obese, and most of us lead very sedentary lifestyles, increasing caloric intake is not as common of a concern as it was back in the 1950s. Nor do most of us have room in our diets for calorically dense foods, like oils. Remember that oil has 4,000 calories per pound, and almost 2,000 calories per cup! That is an entire daily allotment of calories for many people. And drizzling a half-cup of olive oil over a salad or into a pan to sauté adds up shockingly fast. We have been gaining weight for decades, and this has become an imminent threat to public health. Obesity was actually classified as a disease in 2013 by the American Medical Association.

Excess body weight adversely influences human physiology via many different mechanisms and is a major risk factor for CVD, many cancers, type 2 diabetes, liver disease, chronic kidney disease, gallbladder disease, osteoarthritis, sleep apnea, and infertility. It is estimated that 2.8 million people die each year as a result of obesity. Thus, to err on the side of caution insofar as making general recommendations, cutting out oil is a proactive approach.

If you are at all thinking at this point, "Wait! What?!" you are not alone. This was perhaps the most complex argument to understand when tackling the principles of this book. Whenever I told anyone that I was taking the olive oil out of the Mediterranean diet, they looked at me like I was a heretic. And when I indulged in the (literally) hundreds of scientific articles and dozens of books written on the subject, olive oil was (and remains) the main attraction of the traditional Mediterranean diet. We may not be able to solve the question about the proverbial perfect diet in terms of ideal fat percentages or fatty acid ratios, but here is what we can sum up:

1. It is quite possible that the Mediterranean diet is effective in spite of—rather than because of—its heavy use of olive oil. This has yet to be determined.
2. The majority of today's population cannot afford hundreds of calories to spend on oil per day, regardless of what type of oil, with the exception being athletes who burn thousands of calories per day and individuals who struggle with underweight, despite having a vigorous appetite.
3. We do not need olive oil for a balanced, health-promoting diet.
4. Opting for whole food fat sources over oils (olives over olive oil, for example) is ideal because they're lower in calories, higher in fiber and nutrients, typically have a better impact on fatty acid metabolism, and don't confer as high a risk for oxidation as oils.

MYTH #2: THE REAL MAGIC COMES FROM THE RED WINE

Dionysus, the Greek god of wine and fertility, illustrates the duality of wine drinking with his nature. Born from Zeus and the mortal, Semele, Dionysus represents both ecstasy and rage, entertainment and brutality, divinity and mortality. According to tradition, his stepmom, Hera, considered the wine Dionysus created to be a punishment to the world that would inspire madness. Yet wine drinking was extremely common during the time when Plato spoke his truth, and he considered wine to be "medicine given for the purpose of securing modesty of soul and health and strength of body."

Wine in the classic Mediterranean diet is in fact a tradition that merits consideration. Perhaps its health contributions include a plausible lowering of blood pressure, due to its inherent calming attributes. Wine represents the lifestyle choice of slowing down and enjoying a meal, a habit that is helpful for mindfulness and stress management. Further, wine (especially red wine) contains a vast array of polyphenols, phytochemicals known to have antioxidant and anti-inflammatory effects. However, it is questionable as to how large a dose of nutrients can be taken in from a light to moderate serving of wine. Alcohol itself has been shown to have health benefits when drunk in moderation, which is equivalent to no more than two servings a day for men and one serving for women. Health benefits include a possible decreased risk for CVD and type 2 diabetes. *Moderation* is of utmost importance here because drinking more than the recommended maximum is toxic and has the opposite effect on the body's tissues, promoting risk for many cancers, liver disease, and even heart disease. All this being said, the risks of alcohol consumption outweigh the benefits for many people, especially youths, pregnant or breastfeeding women, individuals with liver disease, people with addiction in their genes, and, of course, all those getting behind the wheel to drive. It is by no means necessary to drink wine to reap the benefits of the Mediterranean diet, as the consumption of a wide variety of plants along with the elimination of processed foods and animal products and a great effort at consistent physical exercise and stress reduction are plenty toward the trek to optimal health. If you enjoy a glass of wine, it certainly can be a pleasurable addition to meals that may very well offer some additional benefits when following recommendations.

One serving of alcohol is equal to 5 ounces of wine, 12 ounces of beer, or 1 1/2 ounces of spirits.

VEGI-SIDE

MYTH #3: ACTUALLY, IT IS THE FISH
THAT MAKES THE MED SO HEALTHY

Many people favor fish due to their preferable fatty acid profile when compared to other flesh foods. While land animals are dense in saturated fats, fish are less so. Touted for their omega-3 fats, fish are therefore thought of as the "healthy" meat. This is a perfect spot for a refresher on essential fatty acids—perhaps one of the most complex nutrition issues *del giorno*. The research is rapidly unfolding, even as I type. Omega-3 and omega-6, both polyunsaturated, are the two important groups of essential fatty acids. They are essential because we cannot make them in our bodies, and we need them as structural elements of cell membranes and for growth, reproduction, cholesterol metabolism, immunity, nervous system function, inflammation regulation, and more. Omega-6 fats are easy to find in the food kingdom, ubiquitous in most plant oils and also in corn, pine nuts, walnuts, hempseeds, sesame seeds, sunflower seeds, soybeans, tahini, and wheat germ. Because of their wide usage of oils, processed foods are abundant in omega-6 fats. Omega-3 fats are not so accessible.

The belief that fish was consumed in large measure in the traditional Med diet is false. In post–World War II Crete, Allbaugh concluded that the average consumption of fish, both preserved and fresh, was only six ounces per person *per week* ... the size of two decks of cards or two palms of your hand. In the Seven Countries Study, fish consumption varied between 10 and 60 grams per day with the most fish eaten in Japan by far and little consumed in Crete and Rome. The majority of the ALA in the Cretan diet came from wild greens. Fish intake is reliant to some extent upon proximity to water, having especially been so before transportation was as convenient as it is now. On the Mediterranean Diet Pyramid, fish is set in the upper section with recommendations to consume it a few times per week. In 2011, the global average fish consumption was 38 pounds per year, or 11.6 ounces a week, twice the amount consumed in Crete.

However, fish is not an essential part of a healthy diet and there are good reasons to avoid it, making history slightly irrelevant. Fish are among our greatest sources of numerous environmental contaminants that instill risks that are not worth the easy access to long-chain omega-3 fats. Our oceans have been our dumping ground for centuries. Most tox-

Fish and the Fatty Acid Lowdown

Fatty acid metabolism requires intricate analysis and a fairly healthy under-standing of biochemistry. Rather than get muddled in the details, I prefer to streamline it and recommend further study, if you want to delve into the details. Simply-ish stated, omega-3 fatty acids come in three major forms: alpha-linolenic acid (ALA), eicosapentaenoic acid (EPA), and docosa-hexaenoic acid (DHA). ALA cannot be made by the body and is required from the diet. We use ALA primarily as a fuel source, but it is also used to make more of the more biologically active omega-3 fatty acids, EPA and DHA. ALA is found in these whole plant food sources: flaxseeds, hemp-seeds, chia seeds, leafy green vegetables (both land and marine), soybeans and soy products (e.g., edamame, tofu, and soy milk), walnuts, and wheat germ. It is also found in all of their respective oils and canola oil. EPA is an elongated fatty acid that is involved in inflammation, vasodilation, and nu-merous other physiological and homeostatic activities. EPA can be produced by the body out of ALA and is also found mostly in fatty fish. DHA is the longest of the three fatty acids and is also found mostly in fatty fish. DHA is critical for brain and eye function, is a structural component of red blood cell membranes, and is located in high concentration in the retina, neu-ronal cells, liver, and testes. Many factors come into play in terms of how much ALA to EPA is converted based on necessity, presence of and compe-tition for appropriate enzymes, age, sex, health status, diet, and genetics. Fish convert ALA from their marine algae food into EPA and DHA, making it an indirect source of these nutrients. In other words, fish play the middle fish to bring ALA to EPA and DHA. When people do not include fish in their diet, such as Vegiterraneans, we are reliant upon the conversion of ALA for EPA and DHA. A controllable consideration that influences conversion is eating too many omega-6 fats, which throws off and disrupts the balance. Many people commonly eat a ratio of 14:1 to 20:1 omega-6:omega-3 when we should strive for the ideal ratio of 2:1 to 4:1.

ins from the air, food, water supply, chemical processing industries, and more ultimately end up in the ocean, which then end up in the flesh of those inhabiting it. High levels of heavy metals like mercury, lead, and cadmium, as well as industrial pollutants such as dioxin, DDT, and PCBs, can be present in fish. Radioactive nucleotides are also now being reported in fish due to the 2011 Fukushima nuclear disaster. Cesium and other compounds have been reported in fish near the Japanese plant and also as far away as the west coast of the United States. And remember—the bigger the fish, the more plentiful the pollutants.

Fish oil supplements, now a multi-billion-dollar industry, concentrate many fish into each capsule. These supplements have been found to contain toxins, even if the bottle claims it has been purified or distilled. Fish oil has been recommended as a way to reduce triglycerides and CVD risk. However, in two well-performed studies in 2012,[36, 37] omega-3 supplementation both with oily fish or supplements did not live up to its notorious merit. In fact, taking these supplements was not associated with a decreased risk of cardiovascular disease or total mortality. Thus, not only are fish and supplements made from fish another way to increase your toxic burden, they are simply not effective.

The solution to attaining sufficient EPA and DHA without consuming the toxins in fish or contributing to their pending extinction due to overfishing lies in cautious fatty acid conscientiousness. Here are three ways to optimize your essential fatty acid metabolism:

1. Double the recommended dietary allowance (RDA) of ALA from at least 1.6 grams per day (g/d) for men and 1.1 g/d for women to at least 3.2 g/d for men and 2.2 g/d for women.[38]
2. Reduce omega-6 fat intake to encourage balance. (This is one of the top reasons to minimize or eliminate oils, most of which are high in omega-6, as well as processed foods.)
3. Consider supplementing with a direct source of plant-based EPA and DHA. While evidence does not suggest that supplementation is necessary, it can serve as an insurance policy. Microalgae supplements are widely available now. Taking 200 to 300 milligrams every two to three days is reasonable,[39] but consult with your physician first.

The New and Improved Mediterranean Diet

CHAPTER **3**

The Three C's of How We Eat
Compassion, Carnism, and (Over)Consumption

When I was growing up, I suffered from severe gastrointestinal problems. My parents would take me to urgent care and to see specialists each time I had an attack. I was told I had irritable bowel syndrome and was sent off with fiber powders, laxatives, and medications—none of which helped. It took me about twenty years to finally realize it was the food I was eating that was causing me this misery. Once I switched to a whole food, plant-based diet, all of my symptoms went away, and for the first time in my life, I felt in control of my own health. What boggles my mind is that amongst all of the multiple physicians I saw, not a single one asked me what I ate. Tragically, the medical professional taking an interest in their patients' eating habits is the rare exception rather than the norm. It is absolute truth that you are what you eat. Food that enters your body gets digested, absorbed, and adapted into the tissues and processes of your body. You metabolize foodstuff and it literally becomes you. As gold is melted into a piece of jewelry or a tree is pulped into paper, food is transformed into our cells. From what do you want your body to be built?

We can no longer eat the way we are eating. In order to progress in our quest for the best diet, we need to look back to the past—which we

---

In this chapter you'll learn...

- *The primary distinction between the Mediterranean and Vegiterranean diets.*
- *Why exactly the omission of animal products is healthier for all of us: humans, the Earth, and its animals.*
- *One of the leading causes of chronic disease, environmental unsustainability, and animal cruelty.*
- *How the belief that eating animals is normal, natural, and necessary came to be and is sustained.*
- *The true cost of factory farming.*

explored in the previous chapters—and analyze what worked and what could have been done better so that we can return to health. Perhaps more importantly, we need to look around and recognize what our current state of health is and objectively agree that our devolving diet is at fault. Without question, much change needs to occur in order to evolve and move forward. The health of our bodies, our Earth, and our collective consciousness is precariously perched at the edge of a downward spiral of unsustainability. We can no longer eat the way we are eating. We can no longer suffer the consequences on our health, our economies, our environment, and our psyches. Damage is being done in possibly irreparable ways, and something needs to turn this around. I truly believe that we can completely renovate our current climate and ameliorate the world with each choice we make about what we put at the ends of our forks.

Every single bite either harms or helps us. Our bodies are microcosms for the world we live in. If we put processed, fake, refined pseudofoods or animal products that were raised and produced wrought with stress, terror, and illness into our bodies, imagine what that is doing to us at a cellular level! Well, we don't need to imagine. The answer lies in the Centers for Disease Control and Prevention and World Health Organization health statistics. We are killing ourselves with food. In America, billions and billions of our hard-earned tax dollars are unnecessarily being injected into perpetuating and then treating the ill effects of our diet. We are subsidizing health-damaging foods and allowing fruits and vegetables to increase in price, becoming inaccessible to many in the amounts necessary for optimal health. We are promoting medication as first-line therapy much more often than is necessary. Preventive medicine is still considered "alternative" even though it is enormously effective at avoiding illness and has been used around the world for centuries. Healthcare costs are risking our economic future, and truly, the vast majority of costly chronic illnesses are avoidable. Experts estimate that up to 70 or even 80 percent of healthcare costs could be cut with proper nutrition and a lifestyle modification approach. And yet, nutrition is not supported in healthcare to a large extent and not used as a primary therapy. How many times do physicians actually ask what you eat when you're coming to them for help with an ailment or even for just a checkup?

Politics also play an enormous, semi-hidden role in the foods we eat. Huge money and power from the food industry enable dietary guidelines to be based on financial interests and control policies about what gets labeled and what remains anonymous or unclear to the public. Powerful lobbyists often pay for our nutrition recommendations and accessibility to healthy foods. Nutrition policy is designed at a government level, and the recommendations we are given on what we should be eating are colored by bias. Perhaps more importantly (since direct advice often comes via healthcare practitioner to patient), physicians are generally not taught nutrition in medical school. And if they are, it is at the most basic level, and its importance and relevance are grossly understated. The one medical school nutrition class I sat in on defined what deficiency was assigned to a symptom. For example, when you see a goiter, attribute it to an iodine deficiency; rickets means vitamin D deficiency; and so on. But nutrition is not simply nutrients versus deficiency. In fact, we are seeing more excess than deficiency nowadays.

Dietitians are taught much in nutrition school that is clearly and unquestionably passed down from the food industry. Information I received in graduate school on how to counsel patients included tiny words at the bottom of the page saying, "Sponsored by the dairy council." Had I blinked, I may have missed it. Other nutrition students who perhaps noticed the small print could have easily assumed the recommendations of the dairy council to be expert instruction or the information wouldn't have been distributed in an educational setting. Thus, part of my education as a future healthcare practitioner was infused with paid-for sponsorship. Even the certifying agencies for dietitians and physicians are "proudly sponsored" by food companies that are anything but health-promoting (let alone even safe, by most measures). And most of us aren't privy to the extent of what goes on behind the scenes: That fast food companies, animal product providers, and processed food moguls sponsor medical and nutrition conferences, continuing-education courses, and "educational" resources is not a fact that practitioners speak of regularly.

All we, as consumers, get to judge our food choices by is what we see at grocery stores and restaurants; in ads on television, online, in magazines, books, and other media; and by word of mouth. We are taught minimally about how to eat when we are indoctrinated by the food industry beginning in preschool. We are given guidelines (created by the U.S. Department of Agriculture) to memorize while food-sponsored ads hang on the school-cafeteria walls. Further, in the United States, the school lunch program and breakfast program are paid for and controlled by the government (again the Agriculture Department, not a health or nutrition agency). My expertise is not in food politics, but as a concerned consumer, as someone who educates and counsels people on their health and diet professionally, and as a mom, this is unacceptable, and things need to shift in a massive way.

As a dietitian, my proficiency is in food and its relation to human health. Therefore, my focus is on why the Vegiterranean diet is a path to optimal wellness from a nutrition perspective. However, beyond our health, the impact of our food choices extends to all species that join us on our planet. I have interviewed some of the world's leading experts in fields encompassing sustainability, psychology, and compassion, and I am thrilled to share what they have determined!

Omitting Animal Products and Processed Foods: Better for You, Better for the Planet, Better for the Animals

The distinguishing principle that makes the Vegiterranean diet unique and more effective at promoting long-term health and ideal weight maintenance than the original Mediterranean diet is the omission of animal products. Livestock production and the state of our oceans due to fish and fish oil consumption have clearly transformed the end product. Meat, dairy, eggs, and fish found now do not resemble what we had historically consumed. Being fed unnatural diets filled with chemicals, and living and dying under excruciating conditions causes these animals and their products to have different compositions than did animals and animal products in the past. Thus, not only are modern animal products unhealthful, they are one of the biggest contributors to human disease.

Further, the disastrous, cruel methods of supplying the current demand simply cannot be sustained. We are literally forking the planet and destroying billons of animals a year to meet consumer desires, a practice that we will be forced to end in just a matter of decades, regardless of whether we choose to do so. Not only are our bodies better off without animal products and processed foods, so is our environment.

The primary reason for hunger today is poverty, an unequal distribution of income, and lack of resources. And more people in the near future—eight billion people by 2030!—equals more bodies to feed. Driving up demand like this puts pressure on requirements for land, water, and other already diminished natural supplies. Because livestock is the most resource-intensive food source, we will eventually have no choice but to minimize or eliminate it entirely. The good news is that our food choices make the most significant impact, and you have the power to slow down the devastation with your food selection.

Environmental Impact of Eating Animals

Dr. Richard Oppenlander is a sustainability consultant, researcher, and author whose award-winning book, *Comfortably Unaware*, has been endorsed as a must-read by Dr. Jane Goodall, Dr. Neal Barnard, and Ellen DeGeneres, among others. Dr. Oppenlander is a much-sought-after lecturer on the topic of food choice and how it relates to sustainability, all within the framework of fresh perspectives and critical insights. He also serves as an adviser to world hunger projects in developing countries and with municipalities in the U.S. Dr. Oppenlander has spent forty years studying the effects food choices have on our planet and on us. He started an organic plant-based food production company, operates an animal rescue sanctuary (with his wife, Jill), and is the founder and president of the non-profit organization Inspire Awareness Now. Dr. Oppenlander has written a new, groundbreaking book titled *Food Choice and Sustainability: Why Buying Local, Eating Less Meat, and Taking Baby Steps Won't Work*.

I spoke with him about food and sustainability; here is our interview:

JH: Can you explain how the way we are currently eating is unsustainable?

RO: Most of us are unaware of the enormous impact our collective food choices have on the health of our planet and other species.

Most researchers agree that since the early 1980s, we have been in an "overshoot" mode—now using our planet's resources at a rate of 1.6 times beyond what it can provide. By the year 2030, it is predicted that we will need two full Earths to sustain our current rate of consumption. The primary reason for this overconsumption mode is because of our demand to eat animals and animal products. To better understand this reality, let's further examine the word "sustainable" and then the relevance of specific food choice. Perhaps the most appropriate manner in which to view sustainability issues is with an understanding of what we are *losing* instead of what we *have remaining*. I call this global depletion—the loss of our primary resources on Earth, as well as our own health. When we think about sustainability, we must include concepts that reach well beyond energy or use of fossil fuels.

JH: How do we incorporate these concepts in order to achieve sustainability?

RO: The thought of achieving sustainability, in addition to applying to our own individual human health, must account for other species and with future generations in mind. Our concept of sustainability must extend through many layers—economic, social, ethical—not just ecological—and ultimately must be carried by our choice of foods. That's because the largest contributing factor to all areas of global depletion is the raising and eating of more than seventy billion animals each year and the extracting of one to two trillion fish from our oceans annually, which has become unsustainable to our own health and to the environs and natural resources that support us. The production and consumption of meat, fish, dairy, and eggs are responsible for negatively impacting many aspects of sustainability—land and water use inefficiencies, loss of biodiversity, complicating world hunger, diminishing our own human health, depletion of our oceans and fish, and increased GHG (greenhouse gas) emissions and climate change.

JH: Many make the argument that raising livestock in more natural settings eliminates many of these issues. Nutritionally speaking, there are still no advantages to eating animals. If you take out the antibiotics and feed the animals a diet more closely resembling their innate needs, you are still left with loads of saturated fat, dietary cholesterol, naturally occurring hormones, IGF-1, heme iron, and zero fiber, antioxidants, and phytochemicals.

RO: Eating animals is simply unsustainable *whether factory farms are in the equation or not.* Demand for and consumption of animals is more responsible than any other factor for the following set of problems:

1. Increased risk of the most common degenerative diseases and cancers found in the Western world—which is unsustainable to our own human health
2. Increased healthcare costs and loss of productivity—creating unsustainable economic conditions
3. The prevalence of world hunger (77 percent of all the coarse grain produced in the world annually is given to livestock, which impacts food prices, resource use, policy making, and availability)
4. Depletion of our oceans (commercial fishing has caused the collapse and near extinction of numerous species, loss of coral reefs, and destruction of ecosystems)
5. Depletion of freshwater supplies (nearly 30 percent of all freshwater used in the world goes to livestock)
6. Climate change (30 to 50 percent of all human-induced greenhouse gas emissions are due to the raising and eating of animals)
7. Inefficient agricultural land use causing deforestation, erosion, desertification (minimally, 45 percent of all land on Earth is now being used by livestock)
8. Pollution (our atmosphere, land, freshwater, and oceans are all adversely affected by raising and harvesting animals to eat)
9. Loss of biodiversity (plants, animals, and insects are becoming extinct at a rate up to 10,000 times what has been seen for the past few millions of years)

The principal reason for these outcomes is that raising animals for us to eat is tremendously more resource-intensive than growing plants, and animal agriculture produces more waste, pollution, and greenhouse gas emissions. A given area of land can typically produce 15 times more protein from growing plants than from raising livestock. If used for raising grass-fed cattle or pigs, an average one acre of land will produce 480 pounds of meat while requiring 30,000 to 1 million gallons of water and generating 3 to 4 tons of carbon dioxide and methane. If used only for growing plants, that same one acre of land could produce between 2,500 and 45,000 pounds of food with no pollution, no greenhouse gas emissions, and, in many instances, there is no need for irrigation beyond rainwater. The difference in resource use between plant-based and animal agriculture is literally shocking, particularly when extrapolated to global implications.

Animal agricultural practices have even clouded our perception of the term "sustainable." With less than two percent of the U. S. population eating purely plant-based foods, another aspect of our current diet is the cultural and political perpetuation of pseudo-sustainability—the state of believing a certain food choice is sustainable, when in fact, it is not. Fueled by obvious economic incentives, this state of pseudo-sustainability is fostered by proponents of the meat, dairy, and fishing industries by way of misrepresentation and suppression of crucial information and perspectives related to the benefits of growing and consuming organically produced plant-based whole foods.

JH: What can we do to proactively begin moving forward now that we are in this current state?

RO: Because of this unfortunate phenomenon, it is important for us to begin viewing our food choices and production systems in an optimal or relative sense. How "sustainable" is it to raise and eat ANY animal products in a relative sense as compared to plant-based foods? How can we *best* use our resources? What foods will have the very *least* effect on our atmosphere or climate change? Which foods *best* promote our own human health, and which are the *most* compassionate? The choice, then, becomes much easier to make.

The connection between our food choices—specifically that of eating purely plant-based foods—and long-term sustainability will eventually become critical because it won't matter how healthy we strive to be as individuals if our planet is not healthy. The survival of our civilization may ultimately depend on how we most accurately define the word "sustainable" and then how we collectively choose those foods and agricultural systems that achieve the most optimal state of relative sustainability—organically grown plant-based foods.

Psychology of Eating Animals

When I was a teenager, starving for information about the world and fascinated by food and nutrition, I stumbled across John Robbins' book, *Diet for a New America*. Little did I know that one book would completely transform my life and then propel my mission to help make a difference. Learning about the impact food has on the planet and discovering just how animals are raised and slaughtered shocked me into a completely new awareness. I knew at that moment that I could never unlearn what I had just read and that every decision I made from that point forward came with knowledge attached to it. Ignorance may very well have been blissful, but once I knew, that was it. There was no going back. I felt accountable and responsible for my choices, and I never wanted to contribute to that entire system ever again. However, it was not as simple as I had wished.

As I voraciously searched for more information, for ways to help and be a part of the solution rather than continue to be a part of the problem, I read and read and read some more. The Internet was still in its nascent stage, and the ubiquity of social media was years away, so I was pretty much on my own. I had known one vegetarian in grade school. She was my BFF and I had always thought that the fact she and her father were vegetarians was a little odd. I wish I had pried more to find out their story, but I was too young to really understand the concept. By the time I had discovered it on my own, I no longer had contact with that friend, and I was flat out of any vegetarian resources. So I just went for it and decided to become a vegetarian.

I had no idea what vegetarianism looked like, except for the fact that I remembered my friend often ate peanut butter and jelly sandwiches at lunch. My perplexed parents asked, "You are going to be a vegi-what?!" Clearly, they assumed this was yet another one of my phases. Between my lack of understanding of the how-to and the complete dismay and inexperience of my mom (the one who did the cooking in our house) to cook vegetarian, I took a leap of reckless faith. I ate rice cakes, fruit rolls, diet soda, and granola bars. All I knew was that I was to say no to meat and yes to un-meat.

Several months of eating this way passed, and I did not fare well. My parents were worried, as any caring parents would be, that I wasn't receiving proper nutrition. So they enlisted the help of their friend Kandra, a nurse, to help me come to my senses. They essentially staged an intervention, and we all went out to a steakhouse together. As Kandra told me about the woes of iron-deficiency and lack of protein, my parents had me order my food, encouraging a teriyaki steak with a pineapple ring on top. And then it came to the table. And I was sitting there, faced with all of my idealism, all of my accountability and responsibility, all of my deep passion not to hurt this animal ... and yet that fear kicked in. What if? What if I don't get enough protein? What if I do get iron-deficient? What if animals are being eaten every day because it is the right thing to do? What if eating animals is necessary? What if I am crazy for thinking otherwise? How could I possibly live off of plants? How could eating meat be anything but normal? Everyone does it. And that was it. I was scared back. Terrified, really. How I had wished I could simply call John Robbins on the phone and say, "Help? I don't want to contribute to animal suffering and the destruction of the Earth, but I don't want to be sick. What do I do?"

As I sawed into that first bite of flesh, I may as well have been cutting myself—slicing my will, my integrity, my resolution. And as I put that teriyaki-flavored flesh into my mouth and chewed, all I could see was that cow and how he or she must have had a horrible life and a worse death, perhaps, and that was all to end up on my plate in order for me not to have protein or iron deficiencies. That was the hardest bite to swallow of my entire life. It took forever and ever, and I could not get it down my throat. I remember it to this day, so many years and experiences later. And yet, I did. I ate the steak. Or at least a part of it. And I eventually moved on. I went back to my life, feeling guilty and wrong every time I touched or ate an animal or its derivatives, knowing full well to what I was contributing. It hurt because I knew it wasn't me who was suffering, and yet, it was my fault. And in my heart of hearts, I knew that this was not really necessary. I knew I did not have to consume the flesh of another to thrive. But I didn't know what that meant. Nor did I know how to realize it.

Flash forward many years of nutrition and fitness education later, and I was a personal trainer advising that stereotypical ideal high-protein diet to my clients. I also happened to be working (or trying to work) as an actress in Hollywood and was constantly being told to diet, eat less, exercise more, lose weight at all costs. "If you want to work in this town, you need to lose more weight." Well, as it turns out, eating eighteen egg whites a day and chicken breasts with veggies and not much else, all while exercising for hours to "build muscle" and "lean out," worked. I was doing the right thing. I was thin. I started booking more gigs, even a couple modeling jobs! Studying nutrition reinforced that notion, encouraging ample lean protein and low carbs. Heaven forbid you ate anything high in carbs! My lowest moment was an evening when I was scarfing down a whole bag of blueberry-flavored rice cakes because I was starving and craving carbohydrates. My mom, filled with care and love and only wanting to help me achieve my goals, grabbed the bag of rice cakes out of my hand, smiling and thinking she was rescuing me. I was humiliated. And I was hungry. All I remember of that whole period was the ridiculous lethargy, gastrointestinal agony, acne, and let's just say nasty attitude that I had. I was miserable. Thinner, but awful. My body was falling apart, and I was only in my early twenties. This was healthy?

All the while, graduate school continued to support the idea that we need animal products. Of course it did. The trusted organizations providing us information have a vested interest in us learning that. And learning that with confidence. "How many servings of dairy per day do we need, class?" But I also gained a giant, liberating skill-set designed to enable critical analysis. Along with organic chemistry, microbiology, biochemistry, and physiology, I was taught proficiencies like counseling, research analysis, objective fact detection, food science, medical nutrition therapy, and education. My graduate education was infinite. It empowered me to be able to look for myself—to find answers on my own, to never have to rely on any organization or person to tell me what is healthy and what is not. And it was from that seed that I was able to seek deeper truths. That perspective enabled my biggest epiphany ever. Not only do we *not* need animals for food, but we are absolutely able to thrive without them.

In fact, once I implemented whole food, plant-based nutrition into my practice with myself, my clients, my friends, and my family, I never looked back. And, with that, I found peace. Capital-T Truth. Resolution. Instead of enduring acne, gastrointestinal agony, lethargy, and a nasty attitude, I feel healthy, energetic, rejuvenated. Not only do I read about people reversing their cardiovascular disease and type 2 diabetes with a whole food, plant-based diet, I witness it firsthand with clients. I never saw such dramatic results with my clients before as I do today. Weight loss was so challenging, as food addiction and poor food choices were rampant. Simply maintaining a current medication dose was an appreciated objective. Now, it is not uncommon for my clients to reduce and eliminate medications, to lose weight quickly and without suffering, to increase energy and satiety, and to improve health and longevity. I am grateful for my journey, as I appreciate where I ended up and all that I have learned. When I wrote my first book, *The Complete Idiot's Guide to Plant-Based Nutrition*, my enthusiasm was propelled by the belief that maybe I can be that answer to others who, like me, know they don't want to eat animals, but, like me, don't know how to proceed. Joyfully, that was the response to the publication of that book, and I love that so many people felt the same way.

However, I am mindful that not everyone feels quite that way yet. Without any judgment at all and with a heart full of compassion for everybody, wherever each person may be on his or her own personal journey, I know that our society is simply built that way. I learned about this from Dr. Melanie Joy. She radiantly put into words what I had always felt and why so many people do not feel the same in her book *Why We Love Dogs, Eat Pigs, and Wear Cows*. Dr. Melanie Joy is an internationally acclaimed speaker, best-selling author, a Harvard-educated psychologist, professor at the University of Massachusetts, and founder and president of Carnism Awareness and Action Network (CAAN). I interviewed her about Carnism and the psychology of eating meat.

JH: Eating animal products not only negatively impacts our health and the planet, it also has substantial implications to how we perceive and utilize animals. Can you explain these implications and the impact it has on our own psyche and social perspective?

MJ: One of the most problematic misconceptions about eating animals is that it is a psychologically and socially neutral act. There is a global myth that our food choices somehow exist in a vacuum—that what (or whom) we eat does not impact our hearts and minds or our society.

The truth, however, is that eating animals reflects and reinforces a particular mindset, or mentality. In order for those of us who care about animals to nevertheless eat animals (especially given that we don't need to for our survival), we must block our awareness and shut down our empathy. We must disconnect from the reality that we are eating some*one* and instead perceive ourselves as eating some*thing*. We must act against our core values—values such as compassion, justice, and honesty—and we (unintentionally) end up supporting a global atrocity that has caused more bloodshed than all wars, famines, genocides, and pandemics combined. And the way we are able to do all this is through massive social conditioning that is outside of our awareness and thus outside of our control. We are conditioned to internalize the "carnistic mentality."

Carnism is the invisible belief system, or ideology, that conditions us to eat certain animals. We tend to assume that only vegans (and vegetarians) bring their beliefs to the dinner table. But when eating animals is not a necessity for survival, which is the case in much of the world today, then it is a choice—and choices always stem from beliefs. In short, carnism is essentially the opposite of veganism.

Yet while veganism is easy to recognize as an ideology, carnism is not. That is because carnism is a dominant ideology: it is woven through the very fabric of society to shape norms, laws, beliefs, behaviors, etc., becoming internalized, shaping the very way we think and feel about eating animals. But it is not only because carnism is so pervasive that it remains invisible; the system is actually constructed to keep itself invisible. Carnism is a violent ideology—meat cannot be procured without violence, and egg and dairy production cause extensive harm to animals—and most people would not willingly support such violence were they truly aware of it. So violent systems such as carnism need to use a set of psychological and social defense mechanisms so that humane people participate in inhumane practices without fully realizing what they are doing.

The primary defense of carnism is denial: if we deny there is a problem in the first place, we don't have to do anything about it. Denial is expressed largely through invisibility, and the primary way carnism remains invisible is by remaining unnamed: if we don't name it, we can't even think about it or question it. But not only is the ideology itself invisible, so, too, are the victims of the system. And the victims of carnism include not only the animals, but also those of us who consume them, as we are at increased risk for some of the most serious diseases of the industrialized world and we have been conditioned to disconnect, psychologically and emotionally, from the truth of our experience throughout our lives.

Another carnistic defense is justification, and the way that we learn to justify eating animals is by learning to believe that the myths of meat, eggs, and dairy are the facts of meat, eggs, and dairy. There is a vast mythology surrounding eating animals, but all of these myths fall under what I refer to as the Three Ns of Justification: eating animals is normal, natural, and necessary. And perhaps not surprisingly, these myths have been invoked throughout history to justify other exploitative practices, from slavery to male dominance.

Carnism also defends itself by distorting our perceptions of meat/eggs/dairy and the animals we eat so that we can feel comfortable enough to consume them. We learn, for instance, to view farmed animals as objects—as units of production, or "livestock"— and as abstractions, lacking in any individuality or personality of their own (a pig is a pig and all pigs are the same), and to create rigid categories in our minds so that we can harbor very different feelings and carry out very different behaviors toward different species.

JH: What are the psychological benefits of omitting animal products from our diet?

MJ: When we stop eating animals, we help to free our minds and our hearts. It takes a tremendous amount of energy to remain blind to what is right in front of us, to justify those behaviors we aren't truly comfortable with, to numb ourselves to the truth of our experience. When we stop eating animals, we not only change our behavior, we shift our consciousness. We shift from a carnistic mentality that relies on denial, violence, defensiveness, oppression, and apathy to a mentality that more fully embraces truth, compassion, openness, justice, and empathy. We practice greater integrity in our lives, as we live more fully in alignment with our core values. Indeed, integrity is the integration of values and practices.

When we stop eating animals, we have the opportunity to become active witnesses in the transformation of a violent, entrenched system, rather than passive bystanders who invariably enable such a system. For we are all participants in carnism; our choice is therefore not *whether* we participate, but *how* we participate. When we choose to stop eating animals, we are ultimately able to lead more authentic and freely chosen lives, creating a better world for all beings, human and nonhuman alike.

Even if we do not entirely stop eating animals, or eliminate all carnistic products, by simply supporting vegan values and vegans and committing to moving along the carnistic continuum toward a more vegan lifestyle, we can be powerful allies to the animals and to the vegan movement. Whether as vegans or as vegan allies, we can have the opportunity to one day look back on our lives and feel that when it comes to the atrocity that is carnism, we stood on the right side of history.

JH: Many people who are or are trying to eat a plant-based diet are bombarded with pressure from friends, family, colleagues, healthcare practitioners, etc., and it is easy to question oneself, get frustrated, or simply want peace. What are some effective strategies for handling this pressure and avoid confrontation or discomfort?

MJ: Carnism is structured so as to create paths of least resistance—norms that we are conditioned to follow and which we are chastised for deviating from. Thus, there is often tremendous pressure to conform to the carnistic status quo (though such pressure is diminishing as veganism becomes increasingly understood and respected).

When we stereotype vegans, we portray them in such a way as to discredit their argument: when you shoot the messenger, you don't have to take seriously the implications of his or her message. Vegans may be seen, for instance, as moralistic, picky, self-righteous, overly emotional, militant, flaky, etc.

One of the most empowering ways for vegans to resist this peer pressure is to connect with other vegans, to find a community where they can feel witnessed and validated in their choices. There are many meetup groups, organizations, and online forums that provide such a service. Another way vegans can feel more empowered living in a dominant culture is by becoming educated —learning about the philosophical and psychological foundations of veganism so they can feel more grounded in and better able to articulate their choices to others. It is also valuable for vegans to recognize that the defensiveness they may be confronted with often has little, if anything, to do with them and much to do with the deeply entrenched carnistic prejudice it reflects. When vegans recognize that they are on the receiving end of prejudice, they are less likely to internalize the hostility they experience and are better able to communicate with others about the issue of eating animals and about the bias surrounding this issue. And they are less likely to question the truth of their experience when, for instance, they realize that the doctor who insists they revert to eating meat has studied not medicine, but carnistic medicine—as have all professionals who are the product of the dominant culture.

Compassion

I lost my cocker spaniel, Latte, last year. Latte was my first child. He was a gift from my husband days after my grandmother passed away, just weeks after we were married. Latte was eight weeks old when we found him, and I adored him. He taught me patience, acceptance, and unconditional love. He helped me get through grad school, sitting on my lap as I memorized the Krebs cycle and practiced speeches out loud to him before presenting in class. He sat next to me as I wrote my books, as I went through my two pregnancies, and during all-nighters with the babies. He even photobombed my cooking videos that were filmed in my kitchen, "clickity clacking" all over the sound and trying to steal ingredients. He was my co-pilot and my best friend, as we spent all day long together for twelve and a half years. When he passed away from cancer, my world stopped. His passing marked the end of an era. I had lost loved ones many times throughout my life, but nobody with whom I had had the honor of spending the vast majority of my days. And it was brutal. Every time I looked into Latte's eyes, I saw compassion, vulnerability, innocence. He was non-judgmental, loyal, and supportive. I went from meat-eater to vegan partly because of what I saw in his eyes.

For me, looking into the eyes of an animal reflects the soul and the heart, and a connection is undeniable. When I watch the undercover investigations at factory farms and slaughterhouses, it hurts. I cannot imagine the depth of the suffering of these animals. Modern-day heroes for me are people like Gene Baur, who has been hailed as "the conscience of the food movement" by *TIME* magazine. Gene is co-founder and president of Farm Sanctuary, America's leading farm-animal protection organization. For twenty-five years, he has traveled extensively, campaigning to raise awareness about the abuses of industrialized factory farming and our cheap food system. His book, *Farm Sanctuary: Changing Hearts and Minds About Animals and Food*, appeared on the *Los Angeles Times* and the *Boston Globe* best-seller lists. Here is our interview about factory farming:

JH: The meat, egg, and dairy industries have been forced into extraordinary and excruciating measures in order to meet the current population demand for animal consumption. You've witnessed this firsthand. Can you explain what factory farms are and describe what goes on behind the walls?

GB: Factory farming is characterized by an attitude that commodifies sentient life and regards animals and the natural world as exploitable resources. Farm animals suffer both physical and psychological disorders. They are treated like tools of production, confined in warehouses and denied basic humane consideration in systems designed to maximize short-term profit. They are genetically manipulated for production-related traits like fast growth, but this causes other problems including lameness (because their legs cannot support their heavy bodies) and heart attacks (because their hearts and lungs cannot support the abnormal growth rate). Turkeys have been so profoundly altered that they cannot reproduce naturally so all commercial turkeys raised are products of artificial insemination. The quest to increase productivity through genetic manipulation continues as long as the costs associated with managing the animals' illnesses are less than the profits generated by the animals' enhanced growth rate, or increased level of egg or milk production. Most farm animals live short, tortured lives, confined in stressful, overcrowded conditions—many are packed so tightly that they cannot even turn around or stretch their limbs. To keep the animals alive and productive under such conditions, they are routinely fed antibiotics, which lead to the development of antibiotic resistant pathogens. Still, factory farmed animals commonly succumb to disease, and it is legal for diseased animals to be slaughtered and used for human food in the U.S.

JH: There is a widespread belief that smaller-farmed and/or pasture-raised animals are devoid of cruelty and extreme methods. How accurate is this?

GB: With growing opposition to factory farming, consumers are looking for alternatives, but unfortunately, meat, milk, and eggs sold as "humane" or "free-range" or otherwise as an alternative to factory farming tend to come from animals who are treated poorly. The demand for alternatives is strong, but very few farm animals are raised under non-factory farm conditions, which allows agri-business to sell factory-farmed animal products at an elevated price. Labels are misleading, designed more to sell product than to educate citizens about production practices. The only way to actually know how animals are being treated is to visit farms where they are being raised and slaughterhouses where they are being killed.

JH: And yet these factories and slaughterhouses are kept in secrecy, with laws to prevent people from witnessing what really goes on. You have been rescuing animals at Farm Sanctuary since 1986. What happens to these animals once they are living in conditions where they can move, be free, and be cared for?

GB: When animals first come to Farm Sanctuary, they are commonly suffering from physical and psychological disabilities. We clean and dress wounds, help to mend broken bones and other injuries, and treat them for various diseases and infections. We also show them kindness and work to dispel their fear of human beings. Many heal quickly after coming to Farm Sanctuary. They begin to play and enjoy life and develop friendships, and their individual personalities blossom. They are free to run in expansive pastures and to rest in comfortable barns. Others heal more slowly, and some live with permanent disabilities; but whatever the case, they are all safe and cared for, and they will never again experience cruelty at human hands.

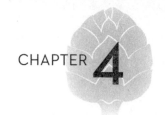

The Veg Ten
Basics of the Vegiterranean Diet

Perhaps nothing is more personal than how and what we eat. Food is so deeply intertwined with our lives, representing culture, tradition, history, love, nourishment, medicine, comfort, and more. With those feelings and experiences, making changes can seem disruptive or insurmountable. But on the Vegiterranean plan, the goal is to ease into it, to enjoy the process, and to do so without judgment. This is a lifestyle transformation, not merely a diet or a quick fix—so a bit of support and guidance during this evolution can make the process easier. Implementing these ten tangible tools is a good place to start. When it comes to choosing meals, no right or wrong exists when foods fall under these ten defining guidelines.

The Veg Ten

1. Pick Proper Packaging
2. Stay Simpler
3. Revel in the Rainbow
4. Focus on Fiber
5. Leverage Legumes and Leafy Greens
6. Favoritize Fats

In this chapter you'll learn...

- *Basic tips and strategies for incorporating the ten tenets of the Vegiterranean diet.*
- *How to prioritize the most health-promoting foods so you can ensure balanced food intake and meet your nutrient needs.*
- *How to get more movement into your daily routine, and sprinkle mindfulness into all of your activities.*

7. Sweeten Selectively
8. Practice Cautious Calorie Consciousness (CCC)
9. Magnify Movement
10. Master Mindfulness

1. Pick Proper Packaging

Contrary to popular belief, we don't eat isolated nutrients. We are not filling our plates with some protein, a side of carbohydrates, and a sprinkle of healthy fats. Instead, we are eating a vast biochemical symphony, built by nature, for nature, in order to function optimally. Nothing represents synergy as clearly as the consumption of whole plant foods. Nutritionism is the belief system that qualifies food based on its individual components. It disregards synergy and the additive effects of a combination of nutrients in one whole food. It ignores the exponentially enhanced value of the interactions between multiple parts and their exchanges within the human body's intricacies. It is the reason people identify their diets as "low fat" or "low carb" or "high protein," even though these diets have not been shown to be the end-all, be-all of ideal eating. It is also the reason that processed food items can be touted as healthy because they only have a certain number of calories or fat grams per serving and are sprayed with a synthetic vitamin to meet the daily recommended dose of vitamin C, for example, despite the fact that they may merely be composed of white flour, white sugar, salt, and multiple chemicals. It is one of the most pressing reasons why, with the thousands of diet fads out there, populations in general are gaining weight and infected by disease, as opposed to building a relationship with real food and connecting it to their lives. We are ostracized from real food when we are specifically seeking out certain nutrients and are dependent upon the nutrition facts label. Labels do not discern between two antithetical foods: an enriched product that was once an intact food, having had its original parts stripped away and then having other ingredients added to boost flavor, texture, and/or shelf-stability versus a real, complete food that had those nutrients in it originally. Although the label may not distinguish between real foods and lab-made foods, our bodies cannot be fooled.

Initially, nutritionism seemed like the magic bullet—that it would help resolve and/or prevent deficiencies. The focus on nutrients served us well, as we have terminated most deficiencies thanks to science and technology. Scientists have greatly reduced the prevalence of diseases like beriberi, rickets, scurvy, and pellagra with thiamine, vitamin D, vitamin C, and niacin, respectively, especially in developed countries. Yet, at the same time, we have also become sucked into a perspective that is based on a pervasive fear of deficiency. And this fear of deficiency has created an over-reliance on nutritionism. But here's the thing: we are seeing more illness caused by *excess* than deficiency around the world. Nutrient-based recommendations need to evolve to food-based recommendations in order to incorporate synergy and to encourage a practical way of eating. This is the premise behind the groundbreaking book by Dr. T. Colin Campbell, *Whole: Rethinking the Science of Nutrition*.[1] During his fifty-plus years in the nutrition industry as a nutritional biochemist, professor, researcher, and more, he recognized the big picture of the damage caused by the reductionism of foods into individual nutrients. Dr. Campbell advocates for an emphasis on foods over nutrients and offers, "If we are truly to understand the meaning of nutrition, its effect on the body, and its ability to transform our collective health, we must stop seeing reductionism as the only method by which to achieve progress and start seeing it as a tool, the results of which can only be properly evaluated within a wholistic framework."[2]

How do we make the giant leap from nutritionism to "foodism?" For this shift in philosophy to take place, it requires a shift in thinking: a move to a macroscopic assessment of what we actually eat—a certain level of seeing from a bird's-eye view. In practice, this change may be as simple as swapping the thought "eat protein" for "eat beans" or retooling the idea "eat a low fat diet" to something more pragmatic like "eat a wide variety of whole plant foods." So, instead of searching for "enough protein" and thinking in terms of "good carbs" versus "bad carbs"—types of misleading recommendations that make nutrition confusing—we need to remember that we eat food and not isolated nutrients. The overall picture matters. Guideline number one is to pick food according to its packaging to ensure adequate nutrient intake—but from whole foods. (It is necessary to note that two nutrients cannot be obtained in sufficient amounts from plants—vitamins B12 and D—which will be discussed in Chapter 6.)

So what's in a package? One of the best ways to demonstrate this is to compare 500 calories of plant-based foods to 500 calories of animal-based foods. This chart is from *The China Study*,[3] titled "Nutrient Composition of Plant and Animal-Based Foods (Per 500 Calories of Energy)." It uses the USDA Nutrient Database[4] and an article on carotenoids[5] since the database does not yet include phytochemicals. The plant-based foods are made up of equal parts of tomatoes, spinach, lima beans, peas, and potatoes, and the animal-based foods are made up of equal parts of beef, pork, chicken, and whole milk:

Plant foods also contain hundreds to thousands of different phytochemicals, which are not considered essential but are perhaps the most effective nutrients at fighting disease (see below). Truth is, our knowledge of phytochemicals is expanding rapidly, as new ones are discovered regularly and their functions and roles in the human body are expanding exponentially. Hence we need to look at the complete picture. A lot more is going on within those foods than meets the microscope. If you com-

Table 1: Nutrient Composition of Plant and Animal-Based Foods (Per 500 Calories of Energy) from *The China Study*[6]

Nutrient	Plant-Based Foods	Animal-Based Foods
Kcals	500	500
Cholesterol (mg)	-	137
Fat (g)	4	36
Protein (g)	33	34
Beta-Carotene (mcg)	29,919	17
Dietary Fiber (g)	31	–
Vitamin C (mg)	293	4
Folate (mcg)	1168	19
Vitamin E (mg_ATE)	11	0.5
Iron (mg)	20	2
Magnesium (mg)	548	51
Calcium (mg)	545	252

pare these two nutrient profiles in the preceding chart, it is clear that both what the plants have AND what they do not have in them are what make them so spectacular. Essentially, the large database of nutrition science consistently shows that the healthiest type of food pattern includes a high intake of fiber, phytochemicals, and antioxidants, as well as a minimization or elimination of saturated fats and processed foods. In other words, both what we eat as well as what we do *not* eat provide the basis for the quality of our overall diet. For the same 500 calories, a meal may be rich in health-promoting nutrients, as well as devoid of all the unwanted ones. So while choosing foods, the packaging must be considered. Both options contain about the same amount of protein, but the plants also contain fiber, significantly more beta-carotene and other phytochemicals, folate, vitamin C, magnesium, calcium, vitamin E, and iron. Plants have zero cholesterol and a better fatty acid profile. Being particular and picking plant-astic packages pays off.

2. Stay Simpler

Leonardo da Vinci is quoted as saying, "Simplicity is the ultimate sophistication." Albert Einstein is documented as saying, "If you can't explain it to a six year old, you don't understand it yourself." And Confucius is purported to have said, "Life is really simple, but we insist on making it complicated." Truth, indeed! Yet, nutrition has snowballed to great complexity as a science, and also as an art when applied to cooking or eating. Explaining fatty acid metabolism demonstrates the irony of Einstein's quote. Aside from science and scholarship and beyond research and healthcare, the complexity of nutrition plays out in how the principles muddle everyday life. Nutrition should be simple and eating should be simple. In fact, the simpler the food, the easier to prepare, and the healthier it is for our bodies. Let's deconstruct the snack as an example. In Crete in the early 1950s, a snack could be tea with bread or fruit. Nice and simple. Nowadays, in the U.S., the most popular snack foods are chips or crackers, laden with enriched flours, genetically modified oils, sugar, salt, high fructose corn syrup, artificial colors, artificial flavors, and/or so-called "natural" flavors, which can technically be any of 500 rather unnatural compounds. Anything *but* simple. To eat simply means choosing foods as close as possible to their original forms—using ingredients in their purest sense—those recognizable food items found in nature. When shopping for food, those items that do not require packaging are optimal. If foods are packaged, the ingredients lists should contain no more than five or so recognizable and easily pronounced ingredients.

A huge, if perhaps unexpected, side effect of eating simply is the progressive adaptation of our taste buds from craving processed and animal foods to enjoying plant-based whole foods. One of the most common concerns clients have when they first come to me to help heal them is the fact that they "don't like the taste of healthy foods." Well, the brilliance of the body includes the fact that most of our cells are constantly regenerating, and we are, quite literally, becoming new versions of ourselves on a consistent basis. This cellular regeneration includes those of the taste buds. In just a few weeks of eating whole plant foods, our tongues may actually become more sensitive to fat, sweet, and salt. Anyone who has ever transitioned from whole milk to skim milk or has reduced sodium intake or has switched from sugar to an artificial sweetener has experienced this dramatic ability of our taste buds to acclimate. We eventually prefer the healthier foods as we learn to dislike the rich and intense ones. I liken this experience to a baby when she is first born. Her taste buds are so pure and unadulterated (pun intended) that breast milk tastes like pure sugar, as it is the sweetest (and the only) taste the baby has ever experienced. With the introduction of saltier, sweeter, fattier, hyper-palatable foods, we develop a tolerance and we become desensitized. Eating calorie-loaded foods that are highly processed with salts, sugars, and fats stimulate the brain to release endorphins, which produce a sense of euphoria. Researchers compare these effects to those that come from addictive drugs. Eating these foods self-perpetuates the cravings and creates a vicious cycle.

Palatable foods are those that have the capacity to stimulate appetite and make you want to eat more. Hyper-palatable foods[7] are those loaded with sugar, fat, and salt, created to stimulate the senses intentionally, triggering a feel-good reward and driving you to want more in order to repeat the experience.

Fortunately, this works in reverse, too. Cutting out processed and animal foods changes the infrastructure of taste expectation, and we soon prefer the whole foods. Sweet potatoes and apples become sweeter; plain steamed leafy greens and brown rice taste salty; oil-free dishes taste perfectly rich. It is as though our tongues have been reborn, and after that, we don't want to eat the way we once did. Those foods simply don't excite our new, evolved taste buds. Personally, I am an ex-chocolate chip cookie junkie. Growing up, my sister and I would hardly get our batter into the oven before eating most of it, let alone leaving leftovers for the next day. I could never imagine my life without cookies. Without even consciously trying to change my love of cookies, it happened after switching to a whole food, plant-based diet. I literally have no interest in dessert anymore. Instead, I go for more kale salad or hummus if I am still hungry. Tell that to my old self, and I never would have believed it! And I have witnessed this experience with many clients over the years. It is a natural and liberating side effect of eating simply.

The number one most effective strategy for eating simply is to cook more. Regardless of what exactly you prepare at home, it will likely be healthier than food eaten out. Society is trending toward eating out more, and cooking is quickly becoming a lost art. Parents are so busy working and/or juggling home-responsibilities and childcare that we are not caring for ourselves in this approach, nor are we teaching our children this essential skill. And so many people are intimidated by the kitchen, uncertain where to begin, how to plan meals, or how to make healthful dishes. Instead of studying and practicing, many of us reach for the take-out menu, dine out, or, worse, eat fast or convenient foods. Here is the secret: we don't have to be culinary masters in order to cook. Simple cooking skills can easily be learned by following recipes, searching websites, and watching healthy cooking shows. One of the greatest gifts we can give ourselves and our families is a commitment to cooking, even very simple foods, and doing so often. The recipes you'll find in chapter 9 have been created with an eye toward getting you in the kitchen—they are simple and delicious.

3. Revel in the Rainbow

A rainbow a day keeps the doctor away and our bodies humming. Vegetables, fruits, and other plant foods provide a broad spectrum of antioxidants, phytochemicals, and abundant vitamins, minerals, and fibers. We get the most nutritional bang for our caloric buck with colorful plant foods—especially vegetables and fruits. Nutrients are considered essential when we cannot produce them in our bodies on our own and require consuming them from our diet. Certain macronutrients, vitamins, and minerals are classified as essential. (We will go into detail about this in Chapter 6.) Fruits and vegetables are loaded with essential nutrients, providing doses of vitamins A, C, E, K, folate, magnesium, potassium, selenium, iron, calcium, amino acids, and omega-3 fatty acids. Plus, an entire additional category of nutrients that are not categorized as essential are at the crux of lasting health: phytochemicals.

Phytochemicals, also referred to as phytonutrients, are nonessential nutrients found in plants. "Phyto" means *plant* in Greek. Scientists have found that although these compounds are abundant, several factors prevent them from being easily quantified and classified. First, so many different types and varieties of phytochemicals are out there that many have yet to be identified. Secondly, levels found in plants vary dramatically according to genetic factors, in response to environmental conditions, and even between cultivars. Finally, assessing how phytonutrients are metabolized and utilized in the human body is difficult because of these added complexities. In other words, if they are found inconsistently in nature, they are more challenging to predict, generalize, and document. Thus, phytochemicals remain the silent saviors, the unsung heroes of our plant food supply. They remain humble, indeed, and go to great lengths to keep us healthy, even without adequate praise. Yet, phytonutrients really aren't made for us, specifically. They are designed for the plants they live within. Plants generate pigments and other chemicals in order to ward off pests, protect against harsh weather, and fend off ultraviolet (UV) radiation, among other purposes. Symbiotically, these same compounds happen to protect our human bodies from a broad variety of concerns. As of now, researchers have identified tens of thousands (possibly hundreds of thousands) of phytochemicals—found largely in fruits and vegetables and other edible plant foods like legumes, whole grains, nuts, seeds, herbs, spices, and teas. Here is a list of just *some* of the vast benefits of these nutrients:

- Reduce cancer activities by blocking the formation of tumors, decreasing the proliferation of cancer cell growth, repairing damage to DNA, and inducing body's ability to detoxify carcinogens.
- Protect the heart by decreasing damage to blood vessel walls, decreasing oxidation of LDL cholesterol, increasing blood flow, decreasing cholesterol levels, and reducing the formation of blood clots.
- Enhance immune function by defending against bacteria, viruses, and fungi.
- Act as powerful antioxidants, neutralizing free radicals that cause cell damage.
- Reduce inflammation, which may very well be one of the primary sources for disease.
- Prevent common eye diseases such as macular degeneration and cataracts and support vision.
- Decrease risk for osteoporosis.

Because each color of the rainbow represents a unique pigment range and broad array of different nutrients, we should aim to eat each and every color every day. On page 70 is just a smattering of the benefits found in the rainbow.

The World Health Organization attributes 1.7 million or 2.8 percent of deaths worldwide to low fruit and vegetable consumption and considers it one of the "top ten risk factors contributing to attributable mortality."[8] Organizations including the United States Department of Agriculture (USDA), American Cancer Society, and Physicians Committee for Responsible Medicine (PCRM) recommend that half our plates be built of vegetables and fruits. Taking full advantage of them means enjoying vegetables and fruits at each meal and providing our bodies with a constant stream of protection.

TABLE 2 Some Phytochemicals Found in Plants, Benefits, and Sample Foods

Color	Phytochemicals	Benefits	Sample Foods
Red	Anthocyanins, lycopene, ellagic acid, flavonols, capsaicin, carotenoids	Reduced risk of cancer, antioxidant, anti-inflammatory, enhanced immune function	berries, cranberries, grapefruit, pomegranates, red apples, red grapes, rhubarb, tomatoes, watermelon, red beans, red bell peppers, chili peppers, red wine
Orange/ Yellow	Carotenoids, flavonoids, bioflavonoids	Antioxidant, enhanced immune function, vision and eye health	cantaloupe, peaches, apricots, lemons, grapefruit, mangoes, nectarines, oranges, papayas, peaches, persimmons, pineapple, tangerines, carrots, corn, pumpkin, squash, sweet potatoes, yams, yellow bell peppers, yellow tomatoes
Green	Lutein, zeaxanthin, catechins, glucosinolates, carotenoids, chlorophyll	Antioxidant, enhanced immune function, vision and eye health, reduced risk of cancer, deodorant, wound healing	green tea, avocados, green apples, honeydew, kiwi, limes, pears, asparagus, artichokes, broccoli, Brussels sprouts, cabbage, cucumbers, green lentils, green split peas, leeks, peas, green bell peppers, leafy green vegetables (arugula, beet greens, bok choy, collard greens, dandelion greens, lettuce, kale, spinach, watercress, etc.), lima beans, zucchini
Blue/Purple	Anthocyanins, flavonols	Antioxidant, anti-inflammatory, anti-mutagenic	Beets, blackberries, black currants, black grapes, blueberries, cherries, plums, purple cabbage, purple carrots, purple bell peppers
White	Glucosinolates, thiosulfinates, catechins	Antibacterial, antiviral, antifungal, anti-inflammatory, reduced risk of cancer	cauliflower, garlic, Jerusalem artichoke, jicama, mushrooms, onions, parsnips, potatoes, shallots, white corn, white tea

4. Focus on Fiber

All of the research articles showing the benefits of plant-based diets and exploring the plausible explanations for the success of the Mediterranean diet typically boil down to two agreeable conclusions: phytochemicals and fiber. These two broad nutrient categories encompass the powerhouses behind the disease prevention and easier weight management abilities that come from eating plants. Both phytochemicals and fiber are unique to plants. Both support our bodies via multiple mechanisms. Well, now that you know why phytochemicals are so phabulous, let's focus on fiber.

If the gastrointestinal tract is thought of as a pipe—which it essentially is, at its simplest—then dietary fiber is like drain declogger, but with added benefits. It acts like a sponge, absorbing toxins, excess hormones, cholesterol, and more, and sweeps them out of your body and through to the toilet. Dietary fiber reduces the risk of cardiovascular disease, hypertension, type 2 diabetes, obesity, and certain gastrointestinal cancers. It improves lipid profiles, blood pressure, blood glucose control, and gastrointestinal disorders such as constipation, hemorrhoids, gastroesophageal reflux disease, duodenal ulcers, diverticulitis, and possibly inflammatory bowel diseases like ulcerative colitis. Fiber promotes regularity, aids in weight reduction, and may improve immune function.[9] Sound familiar? These are the benefits of eating whole food, plant-based and Mediterranean diets. Not only are Americans not eating their fruits and veggies as per minimal recommendations, most people are also skimping madly on their fiber intake, taking in less than half of the suggested 14 grams per 1,000 calories a day. But this can change easily.

Let's break down "fiber" to see where to find it and how to add it to our diets easily. Fiber has traditionally been split into two broad categories: insoluble and soluble fiber. Insoluble means the fiber does not dissolve in water, and soluble fiber does break up in water. All foods high in fiber contain both insoluble and soluble types. Thus, with evolving research,[10] these categories have transitioned into more accurate descriptions based on whether the fiber is viscous or non-viscous and fermentable or non-fermentable, as these qualities are what drive the health benefits.

Viscous fibers thicken and become gummy and gelatinous in water. Found in legumes and oats, viscous fibers promote satiety, normalize blood sugar and insulin levels, and contribute to reduced LDL cholesterol. Nonviscous fibers increase stool bulk and improve laxation. Some fibers act as prebiotics, or food for bacteria in the colon, causing fermentation. Prebiotics promote the creation of short-chain fatty acids (SCFAs) along with gas, which can then be metabolized for use as energy and can also encourage the growth of friendly bacteria in the gut. Fibers that are readily fermentable are found in foods like oats, barley, fruits, and vegetables. Another category of fiber is called resistant starch. Although it is not legitimately a fiber, it acts like one. Because it is resistant to digestion, it also ferments in the colon and fosters the generation of short-chain fatty acids. Resistant starch can be found in foods such as underripe bananas, cooked and cooled potatoes, brown rice, barley, millet, buckwheat, oats, and legumes.

VEGI-SIDE

We have trillions of bacteria found in our gut, known as the gut microbiota, or flora. These bacteria are another example of synergy, as the relationship between bacteria and host is symbiotic. Good bacteria feed off of our waste products and they, in turn, protect us against harmful bacteria. Interestingly, the complex variations in host bacteria profiles very much depend on diet. Healthy bacteria thrive on fibrous food, just as we do. So feed your bacteria as though they were your loving army, setting up camp in your gut, and working hard to protect you.

Surpassing the (bare) minimum adequate intake (AI) for fiber of 14 grams per 1,000 calories a day will help you to improve your gastrointestinal and cardiovascular health, manage your weight easily, and temper your blood sugars. On a Vegiterranean diet, this happens naturally. But here are some ways to boost your overall fiber intake:

- Make half of your plate fruits and vegetables at every meal, especially high-fiber fruits like berries, pears, papayas, and dried fruits and exceptionally high-fiber vegetables, such as artichokes, leafy greens, and squash.

- Include at least a cup of legumes (beans, peas, and lentils) each day. They have up to twenty or more grams of fiber per cup! (More on this soon.)
- Don't throw away the peel of the produce. Fruits and vegetables—organic, if possible—should be scrubbed well on the outsides and the peels eaten for added nutrients.
- Enjoy nuts, seeds, and avocados in moderation (about thirty to sixty grams or one to two ounces of nuts, one to two tablespoons of seeds, or a quarter to a half of an avocado).
- Opt for the whole-grain version of bread, pasta, and rice (brown over white) and include the wholest version—intact grains—like quinoa, steel cut oats, barley, and buckwheat at meals.

Building up fiber intake slowly avoids gastrointestinal distress, as does maintaining a similar amount each day once you've reached adequate intake. Also, drinking plenty of water helps the fiber move through your body.

VEGI-SIDE

5. Leverage Legumes and Leafy Greens

Beans, beans (and lentils, peas, and peanuts) are magical indeed. An excellent source of both soluble and insoluble fiber, luscious legumes help keep the gastrointestinal tract moving and enhance toxin disposal. Legumes help decrease serum cholesterol levels and protect against cancer. They are also key for keeping full and steadying blood sugar levels and, therefore, provide a vital supportive role on the Vegiterranean plate. Used extensively throughout the Mediterranean regions, these versatile, nutrient-dense nuggets can be included in everything from dressings to desserts.

Legumes are a rich source of lysine, an essential amino acid that could otherwise possibly fall short in a vegetarian diet. The amount of lysine in legumes is comparable to that in animal products. In addition to their fiber and protein contribution to the diet, legumes are good suppliers of the minerals calcium, iron, zinc, and selenium. Included in this food

With respect to soy, many people are soy-phobic due to an onslaught of misinformation. Fears of isoflavones, which are the phytoestrogens found in soybeans, include the potential for them to cause hormone-sensitive cancers, cancer treatment disruption, fertility issues, sexual maturity problems, and feminization of men. None of these fears are based on sound scientific evidence. In fact, the research we do have on humans shows a possible protective effect of soy on hormone-sensitive cancers. Soy's isoflavones may even decrease the risk of recurrence or death from breast cancer, and they also may reduce risk for prostate cancer. In 2012, the American Institute for Cancer Research (AICR)[11] and American Cancer Society (ACS) concluded that current research[12] shows no harmful effects to breast cancer survivors or to the general population. One group of individuals that may need to limit soy is those with uncontrolled thyroid issues. The evidence[13] does not show that soy can adversely impact the thyroid. However, for people who already have hypothyroidism and are on medication, soy may inhibit absorption, requiring an increased dose of the medication, but they can continue to consume soy. Due to the theoretical concern about soy instigating hypothyroid disease in those with a predisposition for it, consuming an adequate amount of iodine is an important protection (see more on iodine in Chapter 6).

group are any and all dried and cooked beans, lentils, peas, split peas, peanuts, and whole soy products.

Soy products are great sources of omega-3 fatty acids and plant protein, and fortified soymilk and calcium-set tofu are excellent sources of calcium, among other nutrients. The majority of the evidence suggests moderate intake of soy products—about two servings a day—is recommended to gain the benefits. One serving is equal to one cup of soymilk, half a cup of soybeans, or a third of a cup (one ounce) of soy nuts.

Because the word "soy" covers so many different products, from tofu to soy protein isolate, remember that eating it in its whole form is always ideal. Processed foods in general should be minimized; thus it is the same for soy. Whole or minimally processed soy products include: soybeans (edamame), tofu, tempeh, miso, soybean sprouts, and soymilk. Processed versions, such as soy protein isolate or textured vegetable protein (TVP), found in bars, powders, meat analogues, and other products can be fine in small amounts but should not be considered staples. Further, I recommend opting for organic or specified genetically modified organism (GMO)-free when eating soy. Most soy is genetically modified, unless labeled otherwise. Genetically modified foods have not been shown to be safe in humans.

Enjoy at least one to one and a half cups of legumes a day. Eat them on salads, in soups, and as a base for veggie burgers, bean dips (hummus should be its own food group), baked dishes, casseroles, dressings, and more. (I share how I spread legumes deliciously throughout my recipes in Parte Tre.)

Because leafy greens are nature's true superfoods and filled to the brim with health-promoting nutrients, I recommend you let thy leafy greens be thy medicine and thy medicine be thy leafy greens. Oh yes, they are that fabulous! From fiber and protein to calcium and iron and from folate and vitamins B2, B6, C, and E to phytochemicals, leafy greens pretty much have it all. Chlorophyll, the dark green pigment found in plants, acts as a powerful phytochemical that is used therapeutically to promote detoxification and healing. Many recovery centers utilize concentrated sources of chlorophyll from wheat grass and other plant juices as part of their treatment protocol for seriously ill patients and as disease prevention for healthy ones.

From a culinary perspective, green leafies are versatile as well, offering a multitude of ways to incorporate them into our diets—both raw and cooked. Including both raw and cooked versions of leafy greens matters for three reasons. First of all, certain nutrients are absorbed better when cooked, like the carotenoids found in leafy greens (and other foods like tomatoes). On the flip side, other nutrients like cancer-fighting glucosinolates—concentrated in certain leafy greens (and other cruciferous vegetables)—are better consumed raw. Secondly, when you cook down leafy greens, you can get a whole lot more of them into your body, as they wilt significantly. Finally, many leafy greens contain an anti-nutrient called oxalates in them. These compounds greatly reduce the body's ability to absorb minerals like calcium, iron, and magnesium, and they can potentially build up in your body and promote a type of kidney stone. Soaking and cooking can break down these oxalates. If kidney health is a particular issue, many greens are lower in oxalates, such as arugula, bok choy, broccoli, broccoli rabe, Brussels sprouts, cabbage, collard greens, endive, kohlrabi, lettuce (all kinds), pea greens, turnip greens, and watercress.

Optimally, you'll want to fit in at least two to three servings of both raw and cooked leafy greens every day. One serving equals one cup raw or half a cup cooked. Of course, opting for more raw greens one day and then more cooked greens the next will all balance out in the end.

6. Favoritize Fats

Albeit the cornerstone for the traditional Mediterranean diet, Vegiterraneans eschew the concentrated fats found in olive oil and all other oils, as discussed in depth in Chapter 2. In order to maximize weight management, optimize serum cholesterol levels, and balance essential fatty acid intake, we are sticking with the whole versions over the processed … the whole olives over the oil, for example. Individuals who are not trying to lose weight and who enjoy an excellent serum cholesterol profile may find that including oils in moderation can fit into a healthy diet. Athletes who use up superfluous energy each day and need ways to incorporate more calories into their diets can get away with including healthy oils (like olive oil, hemp oil, or flax oil). However, if you are either trying to lose weight and/or dealing with less than optimal cholesterol levels, a good general guideline is to minimize or eliminate the use of oils altogether. It is the most painless way to cut out hundreds or even thousands of calories a week and to improve your overall fatty acid profile. When eating at home, this guideline is the simplest of all to follow. (We'll learn about preparing oil-free meals at home in Chapter 9.) Eating out is a bit trickier but you can plan ahead and compensate for it by considering overall intake and knowing how to order accordingly (which will be outlined in Chapter 7).

We learned about omegas, ALA, EPA, and DHA in Chapter 2. For Vegiterraneans, diets supporting conversion of ALA to EPA and DHA are essential; the ideal ratio of omega-6s to omega-3s is 2:1 to 4:1. Generally speaking, the best whole fat sources include nuts, seeds, avocados, and olives. Daily essential omega-3 fats can be found in seeds (flax, hemp, or chia), walnuts, soybeans, and leafy greens. Omega-6 fat sources should be enjoyed more sparingly, focusing on foods such as pumpkin seeds, sesame seeds, tahini, sunflower seeds, soybeans, tofu, or wheat germ. Commonly used oils (especially in processed foods) like corn, soybean, safflower, and sunflower oils are high in omega-6 fats, lending to that imbalance between the two polyunsaturated fats. Besides calories and cholesterol, this is another main reason whole sources of fats are preferred. We only need a small amount of fat to meet our recommended dietary allowance (RDA), and we, therefore, do not need to go out of the way to attain adequate amounts. As suggested by vegan dietitian and fatty acid expert, Brenda Davis[14], doubling the omega-3 RDA can be a healthy way to achieve balance. Here is a list of ALA sources:

TABLE 3 A Guide to Meeting Omega-3 Fatty Acid Requirements

Food	ALA Content	Amount Needed to Provide 3.2g ALA for Men	Amount Needed to Provide 2.2g ALA for Women
Olive oil, 1 TB.	0.1 g	32 TB.	22 TB.
Avocado oil, 1 TB.	0.1 g	32 TB.	22 TB.
Kale, 1 cup cooked	0.1 g	32 cups	22 cups
Collards, 1 cup cooked	0.2 g	16 cups	11 cups
Tempeh, 1/2 cup	0.2 g	8 cups	5.5 cups
Broccoli, 1 cup cooked	0.2 g	16 cups	11 cups
Tofu, firm, 1/2 cup	0.2 g	8 cups	5.5 cups
Black walnuts, 2 TB.	0.3 g	20.5 TB.	14 TB.
Soybeans, 1 cup	1.0 g	3.2 cups	2.2 cups
Canola oil, 1 TB.	1.3 g	2.5 TB.	1.7 TB.
English walnuts, 2 TB.	1.4 g	4.7 TB.	3.3 TB.
Walnut oil, 1 TB.	1.4 g	2.3 TB.	1.6 TB.
Flaxseeds, ground, 1 TB.	1.6 g	2 TB.	1.4 TB.
Hempseed oil, 1 TB.	2.2 g	1.5 TB.	1 TB.
Chia seeds, 2 TB.	4.0 g	0.8 TB.	1.8 TB.
Flaxseed oil, 1 TB.	7.3 g	0.4 TB.	0.3 TB.

Eating 22 to 32 cups of cooked kale or 5 1/2 to 8 cups of tofu in a day may be a Herculean task—certainly if it's every day. The solution is to have a little of each of these foods often, especially ground flaxseeds, chia seeds, and hemp seeds. You may also want to complement your food intake with a direct source of DHA and EPA, as discussed in Chapter 2. A sensible 200 to 300 mg dose of a vegan microalgae formula taken every two to three days may be beneficial.[15]

7. Sweeten Selectively

The World Health Organization advises a maximum intake of 10 percent of calories from added sugars in the diet, which is equivalent to approximately 12.5 teaspoons in a 2,000-calorie diet. Plus, they updated their guidelines recently to suggest that 5 percent of calories is ideal. Yet, the average American takes in approximately 20 percent of calories or 23 teaspoons of added sugars a day, roughly double the recommended max! Refined sugar and all of its relatives have adverse health effects, like elevating blood sugar and adrenaline in the blood when consumed. Excessive chronic sugar consumption is associated with cancer growth, diabetes, being overweight and obesity, elevated triglycerides, metabolic syndrome, cardiovascular disease, gout, gastrointestinal diseases, tooth and gum decay, premature aging, depression and anxiety, and acne. Worst of all, it is physiologically addictive. The more we consume, the more we crave. Added sugars hide in everything from breads and plant milks to cereals and desserts, and the only way to avoid these sugars is by staving off anything processed and reading labels carefully. Recognizing ingredient names that are sneaky derivations of sugar is imperative, including:

- the word "sugar" in it, as in beet sugar, brown sugar, cane sugar, confectioners' sugar, invert sugar, organic cane sugar, powdered sugar, raw sugar, or turbinado sugar;
- a suffix of "-ose," like dextrose, fructose, galactose, maltose, or sucrose;
- agave, high-fructose corn syrup, corn syrup, or cane syrup;

- artificial sweeteners, like acesulfame potassium, aspartame, neotame, saccharin, sucralose, or stevia.

Choosing whole food sweeteners while avoiding all calorie-free and added sweeteners is the goal. Calorie-free, or non-nutritive, sweeteners are perhaps worse than other sweeteners due to their powerful ability to perpetuate sugar cravings. Designed by chemists to be super sweet, they provide approximately 160 to 8,000 times the level of sweetness of table sugar. They also promote weight gain via a couple of different mechanisms. First off, a psychological response plays out when we "save calories" by choosing artificially sweetened options. When we feel as if we are taking in fewer calories by picking a diet soda over a regular soda, for instance, it is easy to feel like we can get away with eating or drinking more calories elsewhere, increasing the risk to overcompensate on calories. Further, because our brains sense sweetness from the tongue, the expectation is to receive calories. When no calories come in, the appetite does not get suppressed and the brain is left wanting more. Our highly evolved brain is too smart for us to outsmart it! But we don't need to.

Sugar addiction—and all its damaging health consequences—is broken by sweetening with only whole food sweeteners. Included in that category are the following:

- Dates
- Date paste
- Date syrup
- Fruit purees
- 100-percent-pure maple syrup
- Mashed banana
- Vegetable purees (e.g., sweet potato and pumpkin)

You'll find some recipes for amazing desserts using whole food sweeteners in the recipe section. Of course, as you refresh your diet and revive your palate, you'll be craving refined sugar less and less.

8. Practice Cautious Calorie Consciousness (CCC)

Mangiare di meno is Italian for *hara hachi bu*, "eat less" in English, or *τρώτε λιγότερο* in Greek. At their core, these all add up to a similar concept: eat fewer calories overall to thrive best. Guideline number 8 is called "cautious calorie consciousness" (CCC) *not* because it is a recommendation to count calories and pay attention to calculating numbers. Instead, it is about honing in on an awareness of your personal needs, practicing recognizing true hunger, and eating only as much as you need to satisfy that hunger. This will ultimately result in decreased caloric intake and long-term health. Traditional dieting rarely works permanently, and it leaves out the most important part of the equation: individuality. Most of us eat for reasons other than hunger and end up overeating, especially due to emotions, distractions, and easily accessible, hyper-palatable foods. Eating less using CCC circumvents these challenges.

This feat requires rewiring much of what we already think about weight loss. The science of calories is long-winded and overcomplicated. Yet, we cannot deny basic physics and the first law of thermodynamics, which states that energy is neither created nor destroyed, only transformed. For something that is simply a unit of measuring energy, quite a bit of controversy and confusion surrounds calories. Clearly, we need to consume energy in order to function in the world and fuel our daily activities … even those that go unnoticed, like breathing, thinking, digesting, and repairing. Scientists have gone to great lengths in order to estimate the amount of calories we need for basic survival, in general, as well as for special populations (like pregnant women) or circumstances (like during an athletic event). Measuring exact calorie needs requires special, inconvenient, and expensive equipment so scientists have constructed formulas to help estimate these numbers. Although generalized recommendations are given for how much some body needs to consume, multiple factors hinder the accuracy of those suggestions. Generally speaking, estimated energy expenditures of men are typically anywhere between 2,500 to 4,450 calories and for women 1,900 to 3,260[16]—quite a broad range! Factors that impact these numbers include age, physical activity, muscle mass, and weight. To lose a pound, approximately 3,500 calories need to be cut via reduced consumption or increased activity. With a 500-calorie-per-day reduction, one can theoretically lose one pound per week. However, this application is not a perfect science. It assumes the eating and expending of the same amount of calories each day and demands the counting of calories in and calories out. Plus, the human body strives to maintain homeostasis, putting tons of energy into maintaining a steady weight. Only *we* know our own body. Diets may tout how many calories to eat, when to eat, how to manipulate the macronutrients (fat, carbs, protein) for the ideal path, and/or how often to eat. Yet, the truth lies within. The best gift we can give ourselves is practicing how to tune in and truly, deeply, honestly listen to instincts. Cautious calorie consciousness is a way to turn that attention inward and use subjective scales. It is incredibly liberating and empowering to stop being a slave to the calculator.

Here are three ways to balance energy using cautious calorie consciousness:

1. Although calories count, it's better not to count calories. Instead, self-monitoring may be worth a try. Changes in body size can be measured using the scale and/or assessing how clothes fit. If weight loss is unsuccessful, keeping a very detailed food journal, writing down every bite and sip consumed may prove valuable. Measuring may be precise, using measuring spoons and cups, or simplified, implementing gross estimation. A fist represents about one cup, and a thumb about one tablespoon. On a scale of one to ten, with one being famished and ten being beyond holiday-meal stuffed, a hunger/satiety rating entered before and after eating adds serviceable information. While maintaining an appetite between three and four and then eating only to fullness between six and seven takes practice initially, consciousness but swiftly becomes second nature.

HUNGER/SATIETY SCALE:

1 – Famished, weak, dizzy, unable to concentrate or think of anything but food

2 – Low energy, headache, unable to focus, grumpy

3 – Hungry, stomach feels empty and growls, everything sounds delicious

4 – Starting to feel hungry, but stomach is not quite empty yet, need to eat soon

5 – Neutral, neither hungry nor full

6 – Satisfied, comfortable, can stop eating now

7 – Stomach is full, no more food necessary, food does not taste good anymore

8 – Uncomfortably full, no room left for more food

9 – Very uncomfortably full, clothes feel tight

10 – Painfully full, possibly nauseous and/or bloated, bursting with discomfort

Keeping careful notes and tracking what works and what does not work in a journal is an extraordinary opportunity to control success and figure out the best personalized formula.

2. Hyper-palatable foods designed by chemists and marketing geniuses to stimulate us to overeat should not find their way onto our plates. If we really "can't eat just one," scientists in the lab have successfully accomplished their mission. How can we best avoid this downward spiral? Simply put: don't buy or eat these foods. We have to eat as close to nature as possible, knowing we are up against massive forces aimed at our ability to succumb to those highly refined and processed foods if we do choose to eat them. Relying on the Vegiterranean Food Pyramid (see Chapter 5), we can choose nutrient-dense, calorie-light, satisfying foods to support long-term weight management.

3. Environmental triggers and cues are disruptive but can be played to our advantage. Subtle, yet powerful messages regarding our subconscious food choices infiltrate our day-to-day life. Things like the size of a plate or cup, with whom we are eating, distractions during meal time, and advertisements cleverly displayed on the television or computer in the most subtle ways are all influencing our more than 200 food choices a day. To

stave off these influences, we need to practice awareness and make conscious decisions. Here are some helpful tactics:

- Eating in a quiet, calm setting with as few distractions as possible.
- Using smaller dishes and cups.
- Putting down eating utensils (fork, spoon, or chopsticks) in between bites and chewing each bite well.
- Eating with friends who eat healthfully. Social pressure runs strong and silent. With friends who encourage poor eating habits, choose other non-food activities to do with them, like going for a walk or to a show or taking a class together.
- Trying to avoid watching or reading ads about hyper-palatable foods … or, at least, practicing acknowledging them for their powerful messages and then dismissing them.
- Plating food and then putting away the extras to avoid the temptation of taking an additional serving once full.

9. Magnify Movement

Essentially, the more activity we do, the better (extreme interpretations excluded). Notice how all exercise guidelines from health and fitness organizations are provided in *minimums* with respect to frequency and duration? That is because 24 percent of the population are sedentary and less than half perform adequate daily activity. Thus, experts are forced to encourage the least bit necessary to promote movement. The American College of Sports Medicine recommends a total of 150 minutes per week of moderate intensity exercise, which can break down into five 30-minute sessions. This is the bare minimum to maintain a standard. In the original Mediterranean study, the people who fared so well were very active, walking many miles each day and participating in laborious work. A large study[17] published in February 2014 of more than 90,000 women followed for 12 years showed that the more hours spent sitting or lying down, the greater the possibility of dying from all causes. This was true even in women who exercised regularly! Sitting is lethal, as we are creatures of movement. We need to commit to formal exercise *at least* five days a week for longer than 30 minutes—ideally an hour—and use our bodies consistently throughout every day.

Exercise does not have to be rigid. Whether outdoor or indoor, individual or group, low-impact or high-impact, done at once or broken into segments throughout the day, consistent exercise with variation of form is the key to physical fitness. Cardiovascular endurance, muscular strength and endurance, flexibility, balance, and coordination training are the necessary components to include in a wholistic routine. Mix it up and "just do it!"

- Cardiovascular endurance exercises: aerobic-style classes, bike riding, dancing, jumping rope, kickboxing, plyometric exercises, rowing, running/jogging, spinning, sports, stair climbing, stationary equipment (e.g., elliptical, recumbent bicycle, step mill, treadmill), step or other platform aerobics, swimming, trampoline jumping, walking
- Muscular strength exercises: calisthenics/bodyweight resistance (e.g., calf raises, crunches, lunges, planks, pliés, pull-ups, push-ups, squats, triceps dips); lifting barbells, dumbbells, or kettlebells; pulling resistance tubing
- Muscular endurance exercises: all of the cardiovascular exercises, high-repetition/low-resistance strength training, sports
- Flexibility exercises: dance, myofascial release, Pilates, stretching, yoga
- Balance and coordination exercises: aerobic-style classes, calisthenics, dance, martial arts, Pilates, standing on one foot (then adding closed eyes), yoga

Try these sneaky methods of adding in minutes of movement during the day:

- Take the stairs instead of the escalator or walk up the escalator.
- Move around while talking on the phone (e.g., do calf raises, squats, plies, stand up/sit downs, stretches, or walk stairs).
- Exercise in front of your favorite show.
- Schedule meetings and get-togethers as a hike, walk, or workout class.

- Take movement breaks. Perform a max-out set of bodyweight exercises (e.g., squats, push-ups, lunges, crunches, triceps dips) once an hour at your office, home, or wherever you happen to be.
- Conveniently place exercise reminders throughout your home and/ or office, such as a rubber tubing hanging from a railing, a pull-up bar in a doorway, or some dumbbells by the TV.
- Walk your pet. If you don't have a pet, offer to walk a friend's or neighbor's pet.
- Try wearing a pedometer and aiming for a minimum of 10,000 steps a day. They are really inspiring, and nowadays, plenty of inexpensive options are user-friendly.
- Drink more water to encourage the need to walk to and from the restroom more often. Double bonus: hydration plus more steps!
- Be sure to include fitness that challenges your cardiovascular endurance, strength, flexibility, balance, and coordination as often as possible to keep you vibrant and fluid, ensuring ease in your daily living.

10. Master Mindfulness

Live it up and live fully by practicing savoring the moment. In our hustle and bustle crazy reality where time doesn't always feel abundant, it may seem superfluous to spend time doing less. Yet, we know from the research and from the wisdom of antiquity that sometimes less is more and that this is an extraordinary investment we can make in both our immediate and long-term health. We need only designate a mere five minutes a day to one or more of the following activities—or any others that impart peace:

- Meditate
- Write in a journal
- Spend time in nature
- Practice Yoga
- Listen to or play music
- Draw, paint, sketch

- Read a book or a magazine
- Take a walk
- Practice breathing exercises

Additionally, we can implement mindfulness practice throughout every other part of our day, while eating, walking, or engaging in a conversation, for example. We simply need to tune into our bodies; recognize our surroundings; note how our bodies feel, the temperature, the smells, and the sounds around us; and consider the energy in our fields. Pausing to take a couple of deep breaths also helps us to reconnect and become centered. Thich Nhat Hanh, a well-renowned Zen Buddhist monk and philosopher says, "Life can be found only in the present moment. The past is gone, the future is not yet here, and if we do not go back to ourselves in the present moment, we cannot be in touch with life."

Those are the Veg Ten, the basic tenets of Vegiterraneanism. Simple, easy, compassionate, pragmatic ... like on the Mediterranean several decades ago. If we eat a colorful, varied diet that is as close to nature as possible, move our bodies, and live mindfully, then optimal health, boundless energy, inner radiance, and effortless weight management are sure to follow.

Parte Tre

Vegiterranean
Every Day

CHAPTER 5

The Vegiterranean
Food Pyramid and Plate

A h, the variety of nature's *farmacy*! We can fill our plates with infinite combinations of these fantastic foods, infused with herbs and spices to meet all of our flavor fantasies.

The traditional Mediterranean diet consisted primarily of plants, specifically large amounts of fruits, vegetables, cereals (whole grains), and legumes, very small amounts of animal foods, olives as the main source of fat, and moderate consumption of alcohol. Thus, it is no giant leap to vegan-ize it, as was illustrated in Chapter 2. To illuminate, here are the two food pyramids representing these diets. The first pyramid is from Oldways Preservation and Exchange Trust, originally developed together with Harvard University and the World Health Organization Food and Agricultural Organization in 1994,[1] and the second is the Plant-Based Food Guide Pyramid developed by myself and graphic designer Sherri Nestorowich in 2010 to represent a nutrient-dense guideline for plant-based eaters:

In this chapter you'll learn...
- *All about the Vegiterranean Food Pyramid, which is based on the traditional foods of the Mediterranean but is transferable across the cuisines of the world.*
- *How to put together your own Vegiterranean Plate at every meal.*
- *An intro to carbs, proteins, and fats and their place in the Vegiterranean Diet.*
- *How to get great nutrition while enjoying your favorite flavors.*

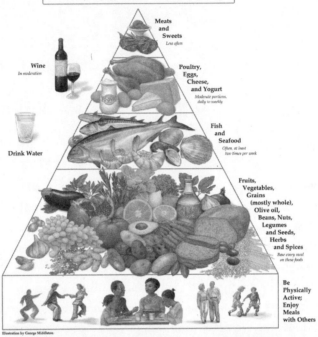

Mediterranean Diet Pyramid
A contemporary approach to delicious, healthy eating

Meats
and
Sweets
Less often

Wine
In moderation

Poultry,
Eggs,
Cheese,
and Yogurt
*Moderate portions,
daily to weekly*

Fish
and
Seafood
*Often, at least
two times per week*

Drink Water

Fruits,
Vegetables,
Grains
(mostly whole),
Olive oil,
Beans, Nuts,
Legumes
and Seeds,
Herbs
and Spices
*Base every meal
on these foods*

Be
Physically
Active;
Enjoy
Meals
with Others

Illustration by George Middleton

© 2009 Oldways Preservation and Exchange Trust • www.oldwayspt.org

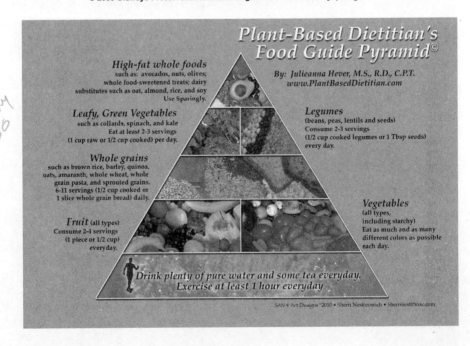

Plant-Based Dietitian's Food Guide Pyramid©

By: Julieanna Hever, M.S., R.D., C.P.T.
www.PlantBasedDietitian.com

High-fat whole foods
such as: avocados, nuts, olives;
whole food-sweetened treats; dairy
substitutes such as oat, almond, rice, and soy
Use Sparingly.

Leafy, Green Vegetables
such as collards, spinach, and kale
Eat at least 2-3 servings
(1 cup raw or 1/2 cup cooked) per day.

Legumes
(beans, peas, lentils and seeds)
Consume 2-3 servings
(1/2 cup cooked legumes or 1 Tbsp seeds)
every day.

Whole grains
such as brown rice, barley, quinoa,
oats, amaranth, whole wheat, whole
grain pasta, and sprouted grains.
6-11 servings (1/2 cup cooked or
1 slice whole grain bread) daily.

Vegetables
(all types)
including starchy)
Eat as much and as many
different colors as possible
each day.

Fruit (all types)
Consume 2-4 servings
(1 piece or 1/2 cup)
everyday.

*Drink plenty of pure water and some tea everyday.
Exercise at least 1 hour everyday*

SAN 4 Art Designs ©2010 • Sherri Nestorowich • Sherrinest@mac.com

These pyramids are not as far off in philosophy as first appears. Essentially, the original Mediterranean diet is a whole food, plant-based diet with a regional identification, a small animal product allowance, and some geographical intricacies. If you simply trim off the upper portions of the Mediterranean pyramid, omitting the weekly and monthly allotments for fish, poultry, eggs, sweets, and meat, only two daily recommendations prove distinctive from the Plant-Based Pyramid: the exclusion of dairy products (described as "cheese and yogurt") and olive oil as a food group. Nutritionally speaking, the Plant-Based Pyramid replaces nutrients like proteins, fats, calcium, and iron found in the animal products from a greater allotment of vegetables, fruits, legumes, nuts, and seeds and displaces the olive oil with whole food fats, which enables a larger possible consumption of fiber, phytochemicals, vitamins, minerals, and antioxidants with fewer calories.

Merge these two pyramids together, factoring in those modifications, and this becomes the Vegiterranean Food Pyramid:

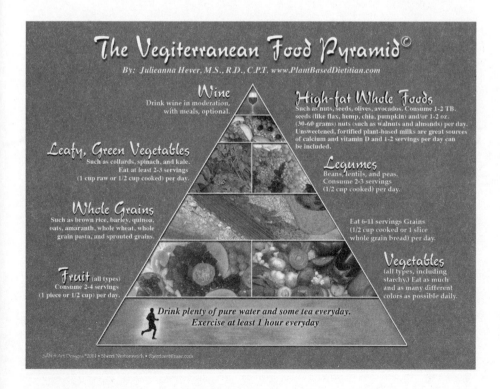

The Vegiterranean Food Pyramid©

By: Julieanna Hever, M.S., R.D., C.P.T. www.PlantBasedDietitian.com

Wine
Drink wine in moderation, with meals, optional.

High-fat Whole Foods
Such as nuts, seeds, olives, avocados. Consume 1-2 TB. seeds (like flax, hemp, chia, pumpkin) and/or 1-2 oz. (30-60 grams) nuts (such as walnuts and almonds) per day. Unsweetened, fortified plant-based milks are great sources of calcium and vitamin D and 1-2 servings per day can be included.

Leafy, Green Vegetables
Such as collards, spinach, and kale. Eat at least 2-3 servings (1 cup raw or 1/2 cup cooked) per day.

Legumes
Beans, lentils, and peas. Consume 2-3 servings (1/2 cup cooked) per day.

Whole Grains
Such as brown rice, barley, quinoa, oats, amaranth, whole wheat, whole grain pasta, and sprouted grains.

Eat 6-11 servings Grains (1/2 cup cooked or 1 slice whole grain bread) per day.

Fruit (all types)
Consume 2-4 servings (1 piece or 1/2 cup) per day.

Vegetables
(all types, including starchy.) Eat as much and as many different colors as possible daily.

Drink plenty of pure water and some tea everyday. Exercise at least 1 hour everyday

S-N-I Art Designs ©2011 • Sherri Nestorowich • Sherrinest@mac.com

The Plant-Based and Vegiterranean Food Guide Pyramids are very similar. In fact, they are almost identical with the Vegiterranean version being based on traditional foods of the Med and adding wine as an option. And here is the subtle, yet vastly important kicker: this plan is absolutely *universal*. An entire, infinite international world of cuisine matches the qualifications for the Vegiterranean diet. Just because the traditional foods of the Mediterranean region are at the nucleus of the research does not mean that you have to stick to the flavors specific to these countries. Asian diets are very similar in food staples, yet the cuisine is dramatically different in flavor profiles. The same holds true with the fare of Ethiopia, India, Mexico, and beyond. The key is holding onto the overall food types. So, what wheat is to the Med, rice is to Asia, and corn is to Latin America. Broad beans in the Med are like soybeans in Asia and black beans in Latin America. Even among the individual Mediterranean countries, the variation of actual foods and recipes is great. Still, the ways of eating all share the same general characteristics:

- Plenty of fruits and vegetables.
- An emphasis on legumes and leafy green vegetables.
- Ample whole grains.
- Moderate amounts of foods containing healthy fats, like nuts, seeds, avocados, and olives.

If you prefer the perspective of the food guide as a plate, see the Vegiterranean Food Plate on the next page.

Overall, the message is to eat whole plant foods with variety, moderation, and balance, customizing dishes to meet your taste preferences.

So Where Do I Get My [Fill-in-the-Nutrient]?

Herein lies the biggest concern of anyone taking the journey from any other way of eating to a plant-based diet and from a nutrient-centered focus to a *food*-centered focus. We will break it down by making our way up the pyramid, defining where we get our nutrients, and learning for how many we should aim. Jumping off the cliff of the comforting and

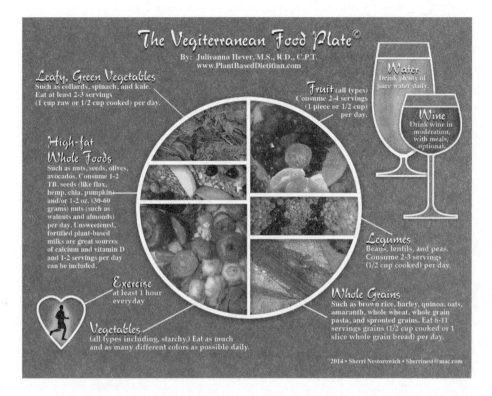

The Vegiterranean Food Plate©
By: Julieanna Hever, M.S., R.D., C.P.T.
www.PlantBasedDietitian.com

Leafy, Green Vegetables
Such as collards, spinach, and kale.
Eat at least 2-3 servings
(1 cup raw or 1/2 cup cooked) per day.

High-fat Whole Foods
Such as nuts, seeds, olives, avocados. Consume 1-2 TB. seeds (like flax, hemp, chia, pumpkin) and/or 1-2 oz. (30-60 grams) nuts (such as walnuts and almonds) per day. Unsweetened, fortified plant-based milks are great sources of calcium and vitamin D and 1-2 servings per day can be included.

Fruit (all types)
Consume 2-4 servings
(1 piece or 1/2 cup) per day.

Water
Drink plenty of pure water daily.

Wine
Drink wine in moderation, with meals, optional.

Legumes
Beans, lentils, and peas. Consume 2-3 servings (1/2 cup cooked) per day.

Exercise
at least 1 hour everyday

Vegetables
(all types including, starchy.) Eat as much and as many different colors as possible daily.

Whole Grains
Such as brown rice, barley, quinoa, oats, amaranth, whole wheat, whole grain pasta, and sprouted grains. Eat 6-11 servings grains (1/2 cup cooked or 1 slice whole grain bread) per day.

©2014 • Sherri Nestorowich • Sherrinest@mac.com

familiar world of nutritionism into unchartered foodism territory requires a soothing blanket of information. Knowledge is empowering and nutrient basics are essential.

Macronutrition Fundamentals

Three macronutrients make up the calories we consume: carbohydrates, proteins, and fats. Alcohol also provides calories (7 calories per gram) but is not considered an essential nutrient. All calorie-containing food can be broken down in these three macronutrients:

CARBOHYDRATES

Carbohydrates (or "carbs") are the classification for a broad range of organic compounds. Simply put, there are two types of carbs: simple and complex. Monosaccharides include glucose, fructose, and galactose, and different combinations of these are found in fruits, honey, and corn syrup.

TABLE 1 Macronutrients

Nutrient	Kcals per Gram	Base Unit	Roles	Good Vegiterranean Sources
Carbohydrates	4	Monosaccharides	Digestible: immediate energy, sustained energy, primary fuel for the brain; Fiber: supports digestion, immune function, cardiovascular health	Fruits, vegetables, whole grains, legumes
Protein	4	Amino acids	Major structural component of all structures and tasks of the body; functions as enzymes, in membranes, as transport carriers, and as certain hormones	Legumes, nuts, seeds, leafy green vegetables, whole grains
Fat	9	Fatty acids	Helps absorb fat-soluble vitamins, minerals, and phytochemicals; major source of energy; provides essential fatty acids	Nuts, seeds, avocados, olives

Monosaccharides, simple carbs, serve as building blocks of other sugars. Disaccharides include sucrose (table sugar), lactose (dairy sugar), and maltose and are found in sugars from cane and beet sources, molasses, maple syrup, dairy products, and malt. Polysaccharides, complex carbs, are formed by large numbers of monosaccharides and can be further divided into either fibers or starches. Dietary fibers are long chains of indigestible complex carbohydrates. Starches, on the other hand, are digestible and provide an excellent source of sustainable energy. Found in abundance in nature, starches are derived most commonly from seeds (oats, wheat, maize, barley, rice, peas) and roots (potato, cassava, yam).

Carbs have been given a terribly bad rap due to fad diets and misinformed ideas. Perhaps the most confusing element is the lumping of all foods high in carbohydrates into one giant group, and referring to it as a food group. Carbs are a *macronutrient*, not a food group. This same standard applies to protein and fat, too. Additionally, all whole foods contain some combination of carbs, proteins, and fats. Worse, carbs (the hypothetical food group) have presumptuously been stratified into good versus bad. A better, more accurate version of this would be to separate carbs into whole versus refined. Therein lies the critical distinction. Intact, whole food sources of carbs comprise the most health-promoting foods on the planet: vegetables, fruits, whole grains, and legumes. Only once these foods are stripped of their wholesomeness do the health advantages disappear and can they be considered "bad." A majority of calories in the Vegiterranean diet come from carbohydrate-rich, intact whole foods. Carbohydrates provide immediate and long-lasting energy and are the preferred source of fuel for the brain. The whole carbohydrate-rich group also include the foods rich in fiber. The recommended daily allowance (RDA) for carbs for everyone over the age of one (except during pregnancy and lactation) is 130 grams of carbs per day. We all need to eat carbs and eat them often.

Glycemic index and glycemic load are scales to measure the blood sugar response to certain carbohydrate-rich foods. Some research studies show using these scales can be a helpful way to regulate blood sugar, especially in people with diabetes, and lower risk for chronic disease. However, a whole food, plant-based diet typically falls lower on these scales anyway and also naturally optimizes blood glucose levels and reduces risk for chronic disease. Consequently, healthy Vegiterraneans need not be concerned about the glycemic index and glycemic load scales.

VEGI-SIDE

PROTEIN

Protein, the other misrepresented macronutrient, plays a crucial role in every structure and function of the body. Our cells, tissues, organs, bones, hair, teeth, tendons, ligaments, muscles, and beyond are composed of proteins. Hormones, enzymes, antibodies, hemoglobin, membranes, and more are created with protein. Protein can also be used as a source of fuel, but the process is not efficient or preferable, like with carbohydrates. Twenty different types of amino acids are assembled into complex sequences and structures. Our bodies can manufacture eleven of these twenty amino acids under most circumstances while nine others are considered essential and need to be consumed from the diet. The six "conditionally essential" amino acids are indispensable when metabolic demands are increased and our body cannot convert adequately.

Here is a breakdown of amino acids:

- **Essential Amino Acids:** Histidine, Isoleucine, Leucine, Lysine, Methionine, Phenylalanine, Threonine, Tryptophan, Valine
- **Conditionally Essential Amino Acids:** Arginine, Cysteine, Glutamine, Glycine, Proline, Tyrosine
- **Nonessential Amino Acids:** Alanine, Asparagine, Aspartic Acid, Glutamic Acid, Serine

All essential amino acids can be found in whole plant foods. When protein from food is digested, it is broken down into its individual amino acids and stored. Then, when it is time to construct an enzyme, muscle cell, or any other protein, the body strings together the amino acids into the appropriate sequence and uses it as needed. Contrary to popular belief, we do not need to combine certain sources of protein at the same meal in order to prevent a deficiency. Even though plant foods contain different amino acid profiles, our bodies are fully capable of storing single amino acids from different sources when we consume a broad range of whole plant foods over the course of a day.

Many people believe that because protein is important, more is better. However, a high intake of protein—especially from animal sources—promotes the risk of cardiovascular disease, kidney disease, cancer, gout, type 2 diabetes, and early mortality. However, most high-protein/low-carbohydrate diets recommend protein levels of up to 30 percent or more of calories, and the average intake in Americans is approximately 16 percent, according to the CDC.

We need approximately 10 percent of our calories to come from protein. In fact, we only need five to six percent of our calories to replenish

TABLE 2 Common Sources of Plant Protein[1]

Food	Protein Per Serving (g)	% Calories from Protein
Romaine lettuce, 1 cup raw	0.6	29
Kale, 1 cup cooked	1.9	27
Brown rice, 1/2 cup	2.3	8
Flaxseeds, 2 tablespoons, ground	2.6	14
Broccoli, 1 cup raw	2.6	33
Kale, 1 cup raw	2.9	35
Broccoli, 1 cup cooked	3.7	27
Whole wheat bread, 1 slice	4.0	20
Quinoa, 1/2 cup cooked	4.1	15
Chickpeas, 1/2 cup cooked	7.3	22
Walnuts, black 1/4 cup	7.5	16
Whole wheat pasta, 1 cup cooked	7.5	17
Almonds, 1/4 cup	7.6	15
Soymilk, 1 cup	8.0	24
White beans, 1/2 cup cooked	8.7	28
Lentils, 1/2 cup cooked	8.9	31
Tofu, 1/2 cup raw, firm	19.9	44

our daily losses. Human breast milk, the single most important source of nourishment for infants intended to support the stage of life where humans grow the most and at the fastest rate, contains five percent of calories from protein. The RDA for protein is set at 0.8 grams per kilogram body weight per day (g/kg/d) for adults; the charts beginning on page 243 show RDA by age.

Whole plant foods provide a plethora of protein in a spectrum of possibilities. Found in everything from brown rice to kale, eating adequate amounts is easy. Some of the protein superstars include beans, lentils, peas, nuts, seeds, and whole grains, but even a starchy baked potato gets almost nine percent of its calories from protein.

DIETARY FAT

Fats, our final macronutrient, also referred to as lipids, are chemically described as either saturated, monounsaturated, or polyunsaturated. All foods contain some combination of these different types of fatty acids, but they all perform varying roles and have unique impacts on our physiology.

Saturated fats (SFAs) are the bad boys discussed in Chapter 2 with the reputation of promoting cardiovascular disease and found in hefty doses in animal products and tropical plant oils. We do not need SFAs in our diet, and less is more when it comes to them. The American Heart Association recommends limiting saturated fats to less than 5 to 6 percent of total daily calories,[2] the amount typically found in a vegan diet.

Monounsaturated fats (MUFAs) are the starring fatty acid in avocados, macadamia nuts, hazelnuts, pecans, olives, peanuts; their oils; and canola, safflower, and sunflower oils. MUFAs have either a neutral or slightly beneficial effect on cholesterol levels. When replacing SFAs, trans-fatty acids, or refined carbohydrates with MUFAs, it may lower bad cholesterol (LDL) and raise good cholesterol (HDL) levels. But, as discussed in Chapter 2, PUFAs may fare better.

Polyunsaturated fats (PUFAs) are typically liquid at room temperature and when refrigerated. Both omega-3 (alpha-linolenic acid, ALA) and omega-6 (linoleic acid, LA) fats fall under this category and are essential in the diet, necessary for growth, reproduction, immune function, inflammation regulation, skin health, cholesterol metabolism, and cellular communication. Excellent plant sources of omega-3 fats include flaxseeds, hempseeds, chia seeds, walnuts, soybeans, wheat germ; their oils; and leafy green vegetables. Omega-6 fats are easy to find in most plant oils and whole food sources include walnuts, sunflower seeds, pine nuts, pecans, sesame seeds, hempseeds, and pumpkin seeds. (More details on essential fatty acid balance are found in Chapters 2 and 4.)

OTHER FATS

Trans-fatty acids (TFAs) are created in a lab via a process called hydrogenation. These partially hydrogenated fats were originally developed to replace butter and lard with the hopes of being a healthier alternative. Plus, they increase the shelf life of processed, fried, and fast foods. Unfortunately, TFAs ended up having major damaging health consequences, dramatically increasing risk of cardiovascular disease. Because the CDC[3] estimates that reducing TFAs in the food supply can prevent 7,000 deaths from heart disease and up to 20,000 heart attacks each year, the U.S. Food and Drug Administration (FDA) issued a notice in November 2013 with a preliminary determination that TFAs are no longer "generally recognized as safe" and is working on eliminating artificial, industrially produced trans fats from the food supply. (Small amounts of naturally occurring TFAs are present in meat and dairy products.) Meanwhile, we need to ignore the nutrition facts part of the food label because "0 grams trans fats" can still legally have up to 0.5 grams per serving. Instead, we need to look to the ingredients list: "hydrogenated" or "partially hydrogenated" tells us to put the item back on the shelf.

Cholesterol is also a type of fat. It is a waxy substance found throughout the body and necessary for the production of hormones, vitamin D, and bile acids that help with fat digestion. Our livers produce all the cholesterol we need, so consuming it in the diet is unnecessary. Excessive intake of cholesterol has been associated with increased risk for cardiovascular disease and, possibly, other chronic diseases. Dietary cholesterol can only be found in animal products.

Phytosterols, also called plant sterols, are plant-derived compounds similar in structure and function to cholesterol. However, these gems reduce cholesterol absorption in the gut, thereby optimizing blood cholesterol profiles and lowering the risk for cardiovascular disease.[4] When combined with viscous fibers, soy proteins, and almonds, phytosterols have been found to be as effective as statins at lowering (unhealthy) LDL-cholesterol levels,[5] but without the negative side effects. All plant foods contain phytosterols, but concentrated amounts can be found in wheat germ, nuts, seeds, whole grains, legumes, and unrefined plant oils such as rice bran, sesame, corn, and canola oils.

Early human diets were professed to be high in phytosterols, unlike the Western diet of today. Plant-based eaters, however, naturally have the highest intake.

VEGI-SIDE

One of the gorgeous examples of the synergy between humans and nature is the fact that whole plant foods contain the perfect ratio of carbs, proteins, and fats, enabling us to simply focus on eating a wide variety of foods we enjoy, so we don't have to calculate, count, or overly concern ourselves with numbers.

Exploring the Pyramid

BOTTOM OF THE VEGITERRANEAN PYRAMID

At the base is daily exercise and water, the two fundamental survival necessities. As previously discussed, exercise and movement should be peppered throughout each day as a consistent habit. What about hydration? Our bodies are composed of approximately 70 percent water as it provides the majority of the composition of our cells. We need to drink water for metabolism, joint lubrication, and temperature regulation, among myriad other roles. The Institute of Medicine's adequate intake for water is about 3.7 liters for adult men and 2.7 liters for adult women per day, from both food and beverages. Hot weather, exercising, pregnancy, breastfeeding, and fever or illness means we likely need additional water on top of that baseline. We should hydrate with fresh water as our beverage of choice. Water is free of calories and, ideally, of chemicals. Drinking the best filtered water to which we have access minimizes contaminants. Plant-based foods also happen to be high in water content, especially raw fruits and vegetables. Still, we should drink a glass of water upon waking and sip a glass of water last thing at night, bookending a day of enjoying water throughout. If plain water seems less than delightful, adding a splash of citrus (lemon, lime, or orange), sliced cucumbers, a couple of berries, or herbal tea can spruce it up. Tea is also included in the base of the pyramid because of its wonderful serving of phytochemicals. A cup or two of green, black, white, oolong, rooibos, or herbal tea (decaf for those who are sensitive or limiting caffeine) are a good foundation for the day.

PERFECT PRODUCE

Instead of whole grains being the food foundation of the Vegiterranean Pyramid, like in the other pyramids, fruits and veggies take the starring role. Besides being jam-packed with phytochemicals, antioxidants, and fibers, all while remaining low in calories, fruits and vegetables also provide a healthy source of carbohydrates and certain vitamins and minerals. They are excellent sources of potassium, folate, iron, and vitamins C and A. Each piece of produce offers a unique nutrient profile, but assessed from a macroscopic viewpoint, fruits and veggies deserve most of the credit when it comes to providing nutrition, influencing each system of the body in a positive way, and staving off chronic disease. Bonus: Fruits and especially vegetables have the fewest calories per pound of any food group. We can enjoy two to four servings of fruits and as many servings of vegetables as we like per day with as much variety as possible. One serving of fruit equals one medium piece, one-half cup fresh fruit, or one-quarter cup dried fruit. One serving of vegetables is either one cup raw or one-half cup cooked. Leafy greens' celebrity status was highlighted in Chapter 4, but note that the Vegiterranean Pyramid recommends including two to three servings per day. One cup raw or one-half cup cooked equals one serving, and this is in addition to the total fruits and vegetables recommendation.

Here are some simple ways to increase fruit and vegetable consumption:

- A serving or two of fruit is a great way to start the day, whether eaten alone, as a fruit salad, or adding berries or apples and cinnamon to cooked cereal.
- A green juice or green smoothie makes a great replacement for one meal.
- A salad and/or soup is a wonderful addition to a meal either as an appetizer or served with the meal. Bonus: Studies show this practice helps us eat fewer calories at that sitting.

- As pasta nears the end of cooking, veggies can be tossed in to soften for a minute or two before straining and completing preparation.
- Sandwiches and wraps taste even better when filled with lettuce, kale, cucumber, carrots, jicama, sprouts, and more.
- Greens make delicious sandwich or burrito wrappers. Big, robust collard greens and cabbage leaves are firm and hold fillings really nicely.
- A bed of cooked greens serves as a tasty base for plating any meal.
- Prepped, ready-to-eat, and within reach is the best way to keep fresh vegetables and fruit in the kitchen.
- Raw cauliflower, baby carrots, celery, broccoli, or other crudité pair perfectly with hummus, guacamole, and other healthy dips.
- Fresh fruit or blended frozen fruit ice cream makes a delectable swap-out for dessert.

Produce is best when purchased as fresh as possible. This means procuring local and seasonal fruits and veggies. Benefits of this include lower prices, more nutrients, better quality, and a lower carbon footprint on the planet. Two great ways to do so are by either seeking out a weekly local farmer's market or signing up to be a member of a CSA, Community Supported Agriculture, where produce is delivered or picked up weekly from a local farm. Basking in the glory of perfect produce is as easy as searching online for a farmers' market or CSA nearby. If you have a green thumb, consider planting a garden. It doesn't have to be fancy or even large, just enough for some favorite staples. Even a mini herb garden on a windowsill helps us to connect to nature and feel empowered. With aquaponics, aeroponics, vertical gardens, and other expanding technologies, growing our own food is becoming increasingly more accessible and user-friendly.

LUSCIOUS LEGUMES

All the legume love was sprouted in Chapter 4, too, along with those lovely leafy greens. Here, let's dig deeper into the details. Two to three half-cup servings a day of these plants from the pea or pod family can be constructed of several different, delicious options. In this pyramid compartment fit all varieties of dried beans and lentils, green beans, snow peas, shelling peas, black-eyed peas, okra, and peanuts. As mentioned, soy products are also included in this category since soy is a bean.

Legumes are inexpensive, versatile, nutritional nuggets that have commonly been enjoyed around the world, playing a central ingredient in most traditional cuisines for thousands of years. Legumes are more conventionally referred to as "pulses," and they have been eaten regularly since antiquity. Lentils require no presoaking, and they cook up quite a bit more quickly than dried beans (especially some varieties) so they are easy to add into a food prep plan. Dried beans should be presoaked and take a bit longer to cook, on average. Because prepping both lentils and beans from scratch tastes better and eliminates any additives, this is ideal (for tips, see pages 186–187). However, with hectic schedules being widespread, canned beans can be a gift and are absolutely fine. Using canned beans saves time and makes for a quick and easy Vegiterranean meal prep. Opt for BPA-free cans and, when possible, sodium-free or "low sodium." Also, rinse them well before eating. If cooking lentils and beans from scratch is an option, it helps us save money, avoid additives, and eliminate chemicals. Plus, they taste amazing!

> **VEGI-SIDE**
>
> Because peanuts are nutritionally more like nuts, they should be treated as such and eaten in smaller doses than the other legumes mentioned here.

> **VEGI-SIDE**
>
> Vegi-Side: BPA, or bisphenol A, is an industrial compound used in polycarbonate plastics and epoxy resins often used as a coating in the inside of metal products, food- and liquid-containing bottles, bottle tops, water supply lines, and some dental sealants and composites. Research has shown that BPA can seep into food and beverages, and exposure may negatively impact the brain, behavior, and prostate gland in fetuses, infants, and young children. Be sure to choose BPA-free cans and bottles!

SPIRITED STARCHES

Traditionally, Cretans and other Mediterranean populations opted for breads made from whole, intact meal as a staple in their diet. Known as "cereals," cooked whole grains such as barley and wheat were regularly included in the meals of these populations. Grains are the seeds of certain plants, mostly cereal grasses, and they are considered whole when the bran and germ are attached and not processed. In this unprocessed version, healthy fiber, fatty acids, and B vitamins remain. Whole grains remain fundamental in the diet worldwide because they are low in cost, widely available, versatile, and store well for longer periods of time. Nutritionally, whole grains provide generous doses of complex carbohydrates, fiber, and other nutrients, making them ideal sources of quick and sustainable energy.

DEFINITION OF TYPES OF GRAINS[6]

- Whole grains include the entire grain seed, or kernel, which is composed of the bran, germ, and endosperm. If the kernel is cracked, crushed, or flaked, the same proportions of the components need to remain, as they exist in the intact grain to be called "whole grain."
- Refined grains have been milled and the bran and germ are removed from the grain, giving it a finer texture, increasing shelf life, and removing fiber, iron, and B vitamins.
- Enriched grains are grain products, usually refined, with added B vitamins and iron.

VEGI-SIDE

A Vegiterranean plate should portion out approximately one fourth to include any intact grains, including: amaranth, barley, black rice, brown rice, buckwheat, bulgur (cracked wheat), corn, farro, kamut, millet, oats, purple Thai rice, quinoa, red rice, rye, sorghum, spelt, triticale, and wild rice. Of course, if you have a gluten sensitivity, allergy, or celiac disease you'll want to opt for the gluten-free grains. Gluten-free grains include: amaranth, buckwheat, corn, gluten-free oats, Job's tears, kasha, millet, quinoa, all types of rice, sorghum, tapioca, taro, teff, and wild rice.

Whole-grain pastas and gluten-free varieties are an easy way to enjoy grains, as are whole-grain tortillas (brown-rice, corn, whole-wheat, and sprouted), whole-grain breads (especially sprouted), and whole-grain crackers. The label should display the 100-percent whole grain stamp, or the ingredients list needs to confirm the fact. Whole grains can be cooked up easily at home, and now plenty of pre-cooked versions can be popped into the microwave or whipped up on the stove in record speeds.

Sprouted grains boast huge health benefits as the sprouting process enhances many of their key nutrients, including B vitamins, vitamin C, folate, fiber, and essential amino acids like lysine, which are often lacking in grains. Sprouting also decreases allergenicity, making them less allergenic to those with sensitivities. Further, research is growing showing that sprouted grains may decrease risk for certain chronic illnesses. Grains are sprouted the same way as legumes so it can be done at home. However, because of their renowned healthfulness, sprouted grain products are already in many major grocery stores. Sprouted-grain products available for purchase include breads, tortillas, cereals, flours, and more.

The general guideline, as in the Vegiterranean Pyramid, is to include six to eleven servings of whole grains per day. A serving is one-half cup whole grains, one slice of whole-grain bread, or one tortilla. This number of servings may be high for some people, particularly those eating less overall (children, seniors, and anyone trying to reduce weight). The best way to estimate portions is to consider one-quarter of your diet from whole grains. These whole grains can also be swapped out for starchy vegetables like potatoes, yams, and squashes or for legumes, as they are high in similar nutrients.

FAB FATS

We've talked a lot about fats from a nutritional standpoint; in short, we need to minimize or avoid saturated fats, emphasize whole food sources rich in essential polyunsaturated fats, and include some monounsaturated sources. On the Vegiterranean Pyramid, whole food fat sources live just near the top. With all of the healthy whole fat possibilities, we only require a small allotment to meet our requirements. Here are some nutritious, delicious ways to include them:

Nuts, known nutritional prodigies, are loaded with healthy fats, fiber, vitamin E, and plant sterols. Excellent for the cardiovascular system[7] and likely protective against type-2 diabetes, gallstone disease, and macular degeneration, nuts have truly reinvented themselves in modern-day science with a continuously supportive track record. Compelling evidence even links long-term nut consumption surprisingly to lower body weight and decreased risk of obesity and weight gain.[8] Nuts happen to be calorically dense, and we only need about one to two ounces (or thirty to sixty grams) of nuts per day to gain the benefits. Nuts are perfect to enjoy in small doses.

Nuts also contain L-arginine, an amino acid that converts into the cellular messenger nitric oxide, which encourages blood vessel elasticity and flexibility and improves blood flow.

Seeds, silent but serious superfoods, are not only the world's most well-balanced source of essential fatty acids, they also contain vitamin E, fiber, plant protein, other vitamins, multiple trace minerals, and phytochemicals, including the antioxidant lignans. Beyond their nutrition, they also serve as amazing culinary magicians. Some examples:

- Chia seeds can thicken liquids into a pudding-like consistency and have become uber popular in dessert recipes of late. Known for absorbing between nine to twelve times their weight in liquid—and quickly—they can also be used to thicken sauces and dressings.
- Flaxseeds mimic eggs when baked, acting as a binder, and they also thicken sauces and dressings. (For info and recipes for egg substitutions for eggs, see pages 177–178.) Flaxseeds need to be ground in order to be absorbed. They can be purchased pre-ground or whole; whole flaxseed should be processed in a coffee grinder or a high-speed blender before using.
- Hempseeds act and taste like nuts for those who may be allergic to nuts, and they are so neutral in flavor that they can secretly be added to almost anything to boost nutritional value.
- Sesame seeds turn into tahini when ground up, which is a calcium-rich powerhouse ingredient for dressings, dips, sauces, and more.

Olives, the Mediterranean's timeless fruit, are delicious as is, without being processed into oil. Rich in monounsaturated fats, phytochemicals galore, iron, copper, and vitamin E, try placing olives on the table as a traditional condiment, adding them into recipes on salad, as a tapenade, or as a healthful garnish.

Avocados are also wonderful sources of healthy whole fat. Half of an avocado supplies a whopping seven grams of fiber, and avocados are also laden with plant sterols, folate, potassium, vitamins C and E, and carotenoids. They make fabulous dip (viva la guacamole) and accoutrements to bean dishes, Latin-style cuisine, soups, salads, and more.

Coconut is a favorite source of fats for many, but it is also burdened by misinformation and confusion. As a whole fruit, coconut can have antimicrobial, anti-inflammatory, and antioxidant properties. However, the primary fat—or about 76 percent of total calories—in coconuts is saturated, one of the few plant sources. Because the type of saturated fatty acids in coconut is different than that in animal products, coconut has been shown to raise the good cholesterol (HDL), which could possibly be a benefit. The jury is still out on any proclaimed overall health benefits, and it is best to use coconut and/or its milk in very small doses. Coconut oil is still considered processed and pure fat. Coconut water, however, is low in saturated fat, high in electrolytes, and acts as a natural, additive-free sports beverage.

Degreasing the kitchen by obliterating oil usage is easier than ever and may awe-inspire a new, healthy, tasty way of cooking. In addition to saving hundreds of calories per day and supporting a healthy essential fatty acid balance, eating oil-free imparts some non-nutritional benefits. First of all, cleaning dishes has never been simpler. Imagine not having grease to scrub! Further, splatters around the cooktop and counters occur less frequently, and if they do, they swipe up easily. Finally, oily stains that destroy clothing can be avoided ... although we still need to be careful with the turmeric and berries. You'll find a few tips for starting out in the Basics section beginning on page 182.

All of the Vegiterranean recipes are 100-percent oil-free, of course, so they serve as examples of how to prepare food in this delicious, healthful way.

THE VINO VERTEX

Vino, or wine, is only the peak of the pyramid if you choose to include it on occasion. It is completely optional and can be seen as either the icing on the pyramid for some or a tier to ignore for many who do not imbibe, especially everyone under the legal drinking age, individuals with health concerns related to the liver, those with addiction, or anyone planning on getting behind the wheel. Keeping wine in the Pyramid makes it obligatory to remind readers that if including wine, please drink responsibly.

SPICE IT UP

No matter what we know about the benefits of eating the Vegiterranean diet, many people may choose to look the other way if it doesn't taste as fabulous as it treats our bod. Not to worry! Not only will transformed taste buds love and appreciate real whole foods after twenty-one days or less, we can also go to town on flavor with fresh herbs, spices, vinegars, and other taste boosters. We can play with delicious Mediterranean classics like rosemary, basil, oregano, parsley, mint, dill, cilantro, lemon, garlic, onion, and fennel—just to name a few of the voluminous possibilities. Spices and herbs are excellent sources of phytochemicals and antioxidants, and literally, the flavor combos have no limits. A good rule of thumb is that dried spices and herbs are about three times more potent than fresh. Thus, one tablespoon of dried in a recipe translates to three tablespoons of fresh. Vinegars offer wonderful, varied tastes for experimenting (while avoiding those with sulfites). Nowadays, fruit- and herb-infused vinegars allow for delectable creativity. Other flavor enhancers include hot sauces, salsas, mustards, extracts, and more.

Nutrizione

Essential Building Blocks of the Vegiterranean

B eyond the macronutrients that we receive from our food, nourishing us with energy to support our bodies' structure and function, other components play critical roles to keep us thriving. These substances—also essential from our diet, but in smaller quantities—are the micronutrients. In this chapter—a micronutrient go-to guide—we'll discuss the nutrients of which we should be mindful and over which ones we should stop fretting. Note that the Institute of Medicine Recommended Dietary Allowances (RDAs) tables for across the lifespan can be found beginning on page 243.

Although it was discovered centuries ago that oranges and lemons could prevent scurvy, micronutrients as we know them today were not really understood until the twentieth century. Initially, the focus in public health was on identifying and solving malnutrition in both industrialized and developing countries, using widespread food fortification, like iodized salt and fortified flour, and initiating dietary standards. Eradicating malnutrition has been an evolving process encompassing politics, science, agriculture, economics, and consistent worldwide efforts. The World Health Organization estimates that more than two billion people worldwide suffer from micronutrient deficiencies, especially in iodine,

In this chapter you'll learn...
- *The myths and truths about dietary supplements.*
- *How best to get critical vitamins, such as B12 and D on a Vegiterranean Diet.*
- *Crucial info about micronutrients: the indispensable vitamins and minerals, their roles, and how to ensure adequate intake.*
- *How the Veg Diet works for pregnant women, lactating mothers, infants, children, seniors, athletes, and those trying to lose weight.*

iron, vitamin A, and zinc.[1] Because it is possible to be overfed and undernourished at the same time, which is one way of perceiving a major part of the modern public health crisis, an emphasis on food quality and nutrient density is crucial. The good news is that by eating whole plant foods, a la Vegiterranean style, nutrients are built in and we can maintain the focus on food over nutrients when eating this way.

As far as we know currently, humans have evolved to rely on food sources for at least 13 vitamins (vitamin A, vitamin B1, B2, B6, B12, niacin, folate, pantothenic acid, vitamin C, vitamin D, biotin, vitamin E, and vitamin K), an essential non-vitamin, choline, and several elements or minerals. These micronutrients are essential for survival and play a role in preventing diseases of deficiency, as well as avoiding exacerbation of chronic diseases.

Some Basic Definitions[2]

Vitamins are organic compounds, essential in very small amounts to support normal physiologic function. Vitamins are divided into two categories based on their solubility. Fat-soluble vitamins require fat in order to be absorbed and include vitamins A, D, E, and K. Because these vitamins are stored in the body's tissues, excess doses can build up and lead to toxicity. Water-soluble vitamins, on the contrary, are not stored in the body. Instead, they are dissolvable in water and eliminated via the urine—so they need to be replenished daily. Water-soluble vitamins include the eight B-complex vitamins, choline, and vitamin C. Because of their solubility, they are more readily destroyed during storage, preparation, and cooking, so including freshly picked, locally grown foods is helpful, as is eating a good portion of total intake from raw foods.

Minerals are abundant in nature, but only a few impact human nutrition. Macrominerals, also known as "bulk elements," are inorganic substances required by the human body in doses of 100 milligrams per day or more. Microminerals, also called "trace elements," are inorganic substances necessary for the body in amounts less than 100 (typically less than 15) milligrams per day.

Vegiterranean Micronutrition

Most of these vital vitamins and minerals are easily available from the Vegiterranean food groups since the options are all nutrient-dense. However, one nutrient is not available from plant sources and another one is hardly available in the entire food supply, theoretically coming via the sun.

B12: The Only Vitamin Unavailable from Plants

Cobalamin, more commonly referred to as vitamin B12, is the one nutrient not directly available from plants. B12 is synthesized by microorganisms, bacteria, fungi, and algae, but not by plants or animals. Animals consume the microorganisms along with their food, and that is why this vitamin can be found in their meat, organs, and byproducts (eggs and dairy). Humans need B12[3] for neurological function, red blood cell and DNA formation, and normal metabolism of all cells, especially those of the gastrointestinal tract, bone marrow, and nervous tissue. Deficiency of vitamin B12 can lead to (irreversible) neurological disorders, gastrointestinal problems, and megaloblastic anemia. People who are at an increased risk for B12 deficiency[4] include:

- People with pernicious anemia, an autoimmune disease inhibiting the ability to absorb vitamin B12;
- Older adults who are not producing adequate hydrochloric acid to absorb B12;
- Anyone with hypochlorhydria, a low amount of acid in the stomach, inhibiting the absorption of B12;
- Those who have had gastrointestinal surgery, like weight loss surgery;
- Anyone with intestinal malabsorption issues, such as Crohn's disease or celiac disease;
- Persons chronically using acid-reducing medications, like proton-pump inhibitors, histamine blockers, or bismuth salts to treat esophageal reflux;

- Vegans who do not supplement with a reliable source of vitamin B12;
- Breastfeeding infants of vegan mothers who are not consuming a regular reliable source of vitamin B12.

The body can store vitamin B12 for approximately three to five years, but after that, with no repletion or with inability to absorb, deficiency symptoms may present; deficiency may also occur with the symptoms lying dormant. Because of this lag time and because serum tests for B12 levels can be inaccurately skewed by other variables, irreversible damage may occur before this deficiency is caught. Therefore, if you're vegan or in any of the high-risk populations mentioned above, you'll really need to keep an eye on your B12 intake.

On the Vegiterranean diet, vitamin B12 may be found in small amounts from fortified plant milks, cereals, or nutritional yeast. However, these are not reliable, adequate means for achieving B12 needs. While claims that fermented foods, spirulina, chlorella, certain mushrooms, and sea vegetables, among other foods, can provide B12 are common, the vitamin is not biologically active in most of these sources. Instead, these inactive forms act as B12 analogues, attaching to B12 receptors, preventing absorption of the functional version, and, thereby, promoting deficiency. For Vegiterraneans or anyone at risk for B12 deficiency, a B12 supplement is an easy, cost-effective insurance policy against any unnecessary problems.

Since we can only absorb approximately 1.5 to 2.0 micrograms at a time, it is ideal to supplement more than the RDA to ensure adequate intake. Many experts recommend a total weekly dose of 2,000 to 2,500 micrograms. This can be split into daily doses or into two to three doses of 1,000 micrograms each per week to help enhance absorption. Because it is water soluble, toxicity is rare.

Here is a handy chart of how to dose your vitamin B12 (specifically from the cyanocobalamin form) across the lifespan adapted from Jack Norris at Vegan Health:[5]

TABLE 1 Proper Vitamin B12 Dosing Guidelines

Age	US RDA (mcg)	Daily Dose (mcg)	2 Doses per Week (mcg)
0 to 5 months	0.4	n/a	n/a
6 to 11 months	0.4	5–20	200
1 to 3 years	0.9	10–40	375
4 to 8 years	1.2	13–50	500
9 to 13 years	1.8	20–75	750
14 to 64 years	2.4	25–100	1,000
65+ years	2.6	500–1,000	n/a
Pregnancy	2.6	25–100	1,000
Lactation	2.8	30–100	1,000

Calciferol (Vitamin D)

Vitamin D, or calciferol, is known as the sunshine vitamin, as it is the only nutrient that we are meant to acquire via the sun. Although vitamin D is classified and treated like a (fat-soluble) vitamin, it is technically a prohormone produced in the skin upon exposure to ultraviolet B (UVB) sun radiation.

Vitamin D is required for peak functioning in every part and system of the body.[6] It is involved in a broad variety of physiological functions including immunity, cardiovascular health, insulin production and blood sugar control, inflammation regulation, and much more. Evidence suggests that low levels of vitamin D likely contribute to autoimmune diseases (including multiple sclerosis, rheumatoid arthritis, and psoriasis), osteoporosis, some types of cancers, cardiovascular disease, and diabetes.

The most well understood function of vitamin D involves its role in boosting calcium and phosphorus absorption in the intestines and reducing its excretion via the kidneys, thereby helping the bones maintain their necessary minerals. Vitamin D prevents bones from becoming soft, thin, brittle, or misshapen as in rickets (in children) and osteomalacia (in adults). Along with calcium, vitamin D protects adults from osteoporosis.

D-ficiency, a Global Concern

Although our bodies evolved to absorb vitamin D via the sun, there happens to be a worldwide deficiency, even in areas where sunshine is abundant. Vitamin D is not widely available from the food supply—especially for those on a plant-based diet. Sources of preformed vitamin D include fish liver oil, oily fish, liver, and, with smaller doses, meat and egg yolk ... all foods best to avoid anyway, with their high concentrations of saturated fat, cholesterol, and other body bashing components. Sunshine and animal sources of vitamin D are in the form of cholecalciferol, or vitamin D3. A second form—ergocalciferol, or vitamin D2—is found in plant sources, primarily from UVB-irradiated mushrooms. Recently, a plant-derived version of D3 was discovered, made by lichen. Dietary supplements may contain either D2 or D3, both of which can be effective at raising blood levels to optimal levels.

Vitamin D started being added to fluid milk, margarine, cereals, and infant formula around the middle of the 20th century. Nondairy beverages, juices, breads, nutrition bars, and other products began fortifying with vitamin D more recently. Although adding vitamin D to foods helped decrease the prevalence of rickets, vitamin D deficiency is still a major global concern. Essentially, if we are not consuming adequate D from the food supply, which is not easy to do, it should be coming from the sun. However there are many variables that inhibit this natural process, including geographical location, season and time of day, environment, natural skin pigmentation, and hours spent indoors. Diseases or conditions impacting liver or kidney function may impact the conversion of vitamin D into its active form. Excess weight also inhibits vitamin D production, while the natural process of aging decreases efficiency of vitamin D synthesis.

Making Sure Your Intake is Sufficient

Total vitamin D intake is difficult to monitor because it can be taken in via sunshine, some natural food sources, fortified dietary sources, or supplements. Sources do not always contain reliable quantities and absorption from the sun is convoluted at best. To further complicate issues, symptoms of deficiency are not usually obvious nor are they always timely. Rickets may appear in babies, but osteomalacia often goes undiagnosed in adults; osteoporosis and other possible consequences of deficiency are not typically overt. Given all this, the best way to keep an eye on your levels is by testing through regular blood tests with your healthcare practitioner.

D-ecisions

If you have a vitamin D deficiency, there are several approaches to consider. Depending on your location, sun exposure, serum levels, age, skin tone, and overall health, sun therapy may help to normalize your numbers. To do this safely, you should spend only a few minutes outside in the sun at peak hours (10am to 2pm, generally) without sunscreen (sunscreen can be applied to protect facial skin and sunglasses worn to protect the eyes). You should leave as much skin exposed as possible—(without making it awkward for neighbors!)—typically just legs and arms. The goal is to start slowly and add a few extra minutes as needed, but never to pink up the skin. Sunburns can promote skin cancer, so you should be cautious. If you are fair-skinned, on average, ten to twenty minutes a few times a week may work. If you have darker skin, excess fat, or are older (over sixty-five), longer exposure is likely necessary. Online vitamin D calculators can help estimate ideal times. If sun therapy is not a viable option for you due to geography, lifestyle, or some other reason, supplements can be very effective. Supplements can also be tricky. The proper dosage should be guided by a healthcare provider, as the difference between building up blood levels of vitamin D to a healthy level and toxicity is a fine line.

The Rest of the Vital Vitamins

Now that we've covered B12 and D, let's look at A, E, K, C, B-complex vitamins, and choline, all of which are effortless to consume on the Vegiterranean diet.

Detailed Institute of Medicine's Dietary Reference and periodic updates can be found online at http://www.iom.edu/Activities/Nutrition/SummaryDRIs/DRI-Tables.aspx.

Vitamin A

Vitamin A represents a group of substances that are essential for immune function, growth, cell differentiation, vision and eye health, gene expression, and reproduction. Consuming vitamin A carotenoids, widely available in fruits and vegetables, provides more than enough A along with that added synergy bonus of the thousands of other nutrients coexisting in the plants. Juicing or cooking carotenoid-rich foods helps enhance their absorption.

Provitamin A and other carotenoids can be found in high amounts in fruits and vegetables that are colored by red, orange, yellow, and/or green pigments. The powerful dark green chlorophyll pigment masks the other colors. Some options include kale, spinach, yam, sweet potato, tomato, carrot, bell pepper, squash, melon, pumpkin, and mango.

Because vitamin A is fat-soluble, it is absorbed best with—you guessed it—a bit of fat. For example, enjoyable combinations include:

- Green salad with tomatoes along with a tahini-based dressing or a sprinkle of nuts or seeds;
- Pasta primavera with marinara sauce served with a few olives;
- Lasagna with spinach;
- Pita with avocado dipped in *sofrito*;
- Baked yams with peanut sauce.

Vitamin E

Like vitamin A, vitamin E is fat-soluble, acts as a potent antioxidant, and exists in several forms in nature. Alpha-tocopherol is the active form nec-

TABLE 2 Sources of Carotenoids

Food	Vitamin A (mcg RAE)
Tomato, 1 cup raw	76
Apricot, 1 cup raw	158
Cantaloupe, 1 cup raw	270
Kale, 1 cup raw	335
Pumpkin, 1/2 cup cooked	353
Spinach, 1/2 cup cooked	472
Butternut squash, 1/2 cup cooked	572
Sweet potatoes, 1/2 cup cooked	961
Carrots, 1 cup raw	1,069

essary for humans. The fundamental role of vitamin E is to protect the body against damage from free radicals. Free radicals are unstable molecules that we come across in our everyday lives, generated from breathing, exercise, cigarette smoke, radiation, environmental pollutants, ozone, certain drugs, pesticides, industrial solvents, and inflammation[7], among other causes. These consistent assaults have progressive adverse effects that accumulate as we age, resulting in oxidative stress that ultimately manifests as disease. In fact, it is currently believed that oxidative stress contributes significantly to all inflammatory diseases and is at the crux of illness and aging. Antioxidants, like vitamin E, can decrease this process by neutralizing free radicals. In addition to its ample antioxidant role, vitamin E also supports heart health.

Excellent dietary whole food sources of vitamin E include sunflower seeds, nuts and nut butters (particularly almonds), peanuts and peanut butter, avocados, wheat germ, and leafy green vegetables.

Vitamin K

The last of the fat-soluble vitamins was named after the German word "koagulation" because of its role in helping blood to clot, or coagulate. Vitamin K helps regulate coagulation so that wounds can heal properly and also to prevent hemorrhaging. It also supports bone metabolism.

When taking the blood-thinning medication Warfarin (brand name is Coumadin), vitamin K activity is decreased intentionally, to prevent clotting which can lead to heart attacks, strokes, pulmonary embolism, or deep vein thrombosis in people at high risk. Maintaining a *consistent* intake of vitamin K-rich foods while taking the prescribed dose of Warfarin is critical for the drug to work properly. Because these foods are health-promoting and support chronic disease risk, speak to your physician about maximizing your intake and ensuring proper dosage of the medication.

Two forms of vitamin K are found in nature. Vitamin K1 comes from plants and is the predominant form found in the diet. Vitamin K2 refers to a family of compounds, which are synthesized in our intestines by bacteria and are found in animal products, too. Although deficiency is rare due to the abundance of vitamin K in dietary sources, it can occur in people with malabsorption, those taking anticoagulant drugs, someone with liver disease, or newborn babies who are exclusively breast-fed and did not receive their initial injections at birth. Deficiency can lead to impaired bone mineral density and compromised blood clotting, evident by bruising or bleeding.

The best sources include leafy green vegetables—especially kale and spinach, as well as parsley, broccoli, Brussels sprouts, cabbage, and asparagus.

Vitamin C

Also known as ascorbic acid, vitamin C is a water-soluble vitamin. Famous for its talents in enhancing immune function and as the victor in curing scurvy in sailors during long journeys at sea, this important nutrient does so much more. Vitamin C—like vitamins A and E and selenium—is a forceful antioxidant.[8] Vitamin C also helps produce collagen, L-carnitine, and norepinephrine and enhances the absorption of iron.

Getting adequate vitamin C can easily be accomplished by meeting the bare minimum daily requirement of just five servings of fruits and vegetables a day. Vegiterranean foods chock-full of C include tropical fruits (papaya, guava, mango, and pineapple), citrus fruits (oranges, grapefruit, tangerines, lemons, and limes), kiwi, berries (strawberries, blackberries, and raspberries), bell peppers, broccoli, Brussels sprouts, leafy greens, tomatoes, cauliflower, and melons.

Bountiful B's

The eight known B vitamins plus choline—which tends to get lumped together with the B's even though it is not technically a vitamin—all are coenzymes involved in various aspects of energy metabolism. Because they are all water-soluble, they are not stored in considerable quantities and, therefore, need to be replenished daily. Vitamin B12 is the only nutrient not reliable from plant sources—we already covered that one—but here are some facts about the other plant-abundant B's.

Thiamin (Vitamin B1)

Thiamin, also spelled as thiamine, is one of the first recognized vitamins. Deficiency of thiamin is called beriberi, a disease that causes weakness, pain, mental confusion, and other neurologic and cardiovascular dysfunction. Alcoholics are at a high risk for thiamin deficiency—a condition specifically known as Wernicke-Korsakoff syndrome—due to decreased intake, compromised absorption, and increased demand of the nutrient. Deficiency can also occur in populations who consume polished (milled or refined) rice since the thiamin is removed with the bran. Dietary sources of thiamin include nutritional yeast, fortified cereals and plant milks, whole grains like quinoa, brown rice, oats, and barley, legumes, nutritional yeast, brewer's yeast, and sunflower seeds.

Riboflavin (Vitamin B2)

Another essential coenzyme, riboflavin plays more of a supporting role in energy metabolism, assisting in antioxidant activity and red blood cell formation. Riboflavin deficiency typically occurs in combination with a deficiency in other B vitamins, and when it does occur, it typically presents as mouth sores, cracks on the outside of the lips, a swollen tongue or mouth, or inflamed and reddened skin.

Riboflavin is easily destroyed by sunlight but is stable in heat, oxygen, and acid. Fun fact: Riboflavin is the nutrient that gets credit for turning urine fluorescent yellow. Excellent food sources include nutritional yeast, fortified cereals and plant milks, buckwheat, quinoa, soybeans, mushrooms, leafy greens, asparagus, avocados, and almonds.

Niacin (Vitamin B3)

Similar to the other B-complex nutrients, niacin is a coenzyme in the processes of converting food into usable energy and in antioxidant activities. In high (therapeutic) doses, niacin improves serum cholesterol levels by increasing HDL cholesterol and improving overall profile, which is why it is often used in combination with other lipid-lowering medications in high-risk people. Niacin also supports the health of the skin, gastrointestinal tract, and nervous system, which is why pellagra, the disease associated with niacin deficiency, is characterized by symptoms that impact these systems. Symptoms of niacin deficiency include "the three D's:" dermatitis (skin inflammation), diarrhea, and dementia. Niacin deficiency is found in people with overall malnutrition and poor absorption. Dietary sources include nutritional yeast, fortified cereals and plant milks, legumes, peanuts and peanut butter, brown rice, barley, tahini, tempeh, mushrooms, and potatoes.

Pantothenic acid (Vitamin B5)

Interestingly, the nutrient pantothenic acid derives its name from the Greek word *pantothen*, which means "from every side" or "from everywhere." It is the rarest nutrient deficiency since pantothenic acid can be found widely distributed in the food supply. Also an essential coenzyme, pantothenic acid helps generate energy from fats, proteins, and carbohydrates; helps synthesize essential fats, cholesterol, steroid hormones, acetylcholine, melatonin, and heme, a component of hemoglobin; and participates in nerve transmission. Exceptionally high sources include nutritional yeast, avocados, mushrooms, lentils, split peas, broccoli, sweet potatoes, and cauliflower.

Pyridoxine (Vitamin B6)

Another coenzyme essential in the diet, vitamin B6 plays a crucial role in the function of at least 100 different enzymes, mostly related to protein metabolism. B6 contributes to energy release, neurotransmitter synthesis, red blood cell formation and utility, steroid hormone function, and the synthesis of nucleic acids (DNA and RNA). Vitamin B6 also assists in normal immune function.

Deficiency in vitamin B6 can be seen in alcoholics due to both impaired metabolism and inadequate intake. Other at-risk people include those eating a diet high in refined foods, people with malabsorptive conditions or autoimmune disorders, and individuals on certain medications that may interfere with absorption. Some sources of vitamin B6 are nutritional yeast, fortified cereals, chickpeas, sweet potatoes, potatoes, bananas, avocados, soy products, spinach, legumes, and squash.

Biotin (Vitamin B7)

Biotin participates in the metabolism of carbohydrates, fats, and proteins for energy. Deficiency in this nutrient is exceedingly rare, found mostly in people who are generally malnourished or not consuming enough calories, but also in those on prolonged intravenous feedings without supplementation and people who consume raw egg whites over a period of time. Deficiency symptoms include anorexia, hair loss, scaly red rash, or neurological dysfunction. Biotin can be found in nutritional yeast, oat bran, oatmeal, peanuts and peanut butter, almonds, sweet potatoes, onions, tomatoes, carrots, avocados, and walnuts.

Folate (Vitamin B9)

Two of the primary roles of folate are acting as a coenzyme in the synthesis and protection of nucleic acids (DNA and RNA) and in amino acid metabolism. For most people, folate deficiency is uncommon, but when it does happen, it coexists with other deficiencies, alcoholism, or malabsorption disorders. Megaloblastic anemia can be caused by either folate or vitamin B12 deficiency. Folate is critical during the initial stages of pregnancy, preventing neural tube defects, premature birth, and low birth weight. Women of childbearing age are advised to consume adequate folate attentively since it is the first few weeks that are most imperative and some women are not aware they are pregnant until further along.

While dietary folate may be protective against certain cancers, high doses of the supplemental or synthetic version—folic acid—has been shown to promote the growth of cancer. So whole food sources of folate should be included in the diet over synthetic folic acid from supplements or fortified foods whenever possible. Fortunately, folate is found widely in the food supply. Appropriately, the root of the words "folate" or "folic acid" comes from the Latin word *folium*, which means "leaf." Folate can be found in hefty doses in leaves like spinach, kale, and collard greens, along with broccoli, asparagus, Brussels sprouts, lentils, beans, split peas, peanuts and peanut butter, soy products, avocados, oranges, cantaloupe, sunflower seeds, and grapefruit.

VEGI-SIDE

Folate is the naturally occurring vitamin version found in food while folic acid is synthetic and used in supplements and fortified foods.

Choline

Choline tends to be grouped together with B vitamins even though it is not defined as a vitamin. It is, however, considered essential in the diet. Our bodies can produce choline as long as our intake of vitamin B12, folate, and methionine[9] is sufficient. Choline plays a role in memory and muscle control. Plant sources include Brussels sprouts, broccoli, beans, soy products, peanuts and peanut butter, and quinoa.

Major Minerals

Although many minerals play a role in our dietary health, there are some that require special consideration: calcium, iodine, iron, and zinc. But first, here are some general notes about minerals: Their absorption in the body can be affected by cooking and some interfering antinutrients (like phytates). It's also interesting to note that if the body needs more of these minerals, it will tend to absorb more. If levels are already up to par, it will likely excrete the excess. Minding minerals is as simple as following these guidelines:

- A good portion of total calories should come from raw foods.
- A wide variety of different foods should be emphasized.
- Consumption of the liquids in which food were cooked provides any nutrients that leeched out of the foods during cooking.
- Blending, juicing, soaking, sprouting, fermenting, and leavening are techniques that help to release nutrients such as calcium, iron, magnesium, and zinc from phytates to help absorption.[10]

Calcium

As the most abundant mineral in the human body, 99 percent of calcium is stored in the bones and teeth with the remaining percentage circulating in the blood and tissues. In addition to playing an essential role in bone and tooth formation, calcium is also involved in blood clotting, nerve transmission, muscle contraction, intracellular signaling, and the secretion of hormones and enzymes.

Throughout the lifespan, adequate intake dietary recommendations fluctuate. Calcium can be consumed directly from the vast variety of foods that boast healthy levels, like leafy green vegetables (yes, they win again), especially bok choy, broccoli, napa cabbage, collard greens, dandelion greens, kale, turnip greens, and watercress. Other food sources loaded with calcium include fortified plant milks, calcium-set tofu, dried figs, sesame seeds and tahini, tempeh, almonds and almond butter, oranges, sweet potatoes, and beans.

Regardless of how much calcium is consumed, the key issue is how much is actually *absorbed*. Many variables impact calcium levels via absorption or excretion including:

- Amount consumed. We can only absorb approximately 500 milligrams at a time, and absorption decreases as calcium intake increases.
- Age. Calcium absorption is highest in infants and children, as they are rapidly growing bone. Absorption capability progressively decreases as we age.
- Phytates found in whole grains, beans, seeds, nuts, and wheat bran can bind to calcium (and other minerals) and inhibit absorption. Soaking, sprouting, leavening, and fermenting helps improve the absorption.
- Oxalates are substances found in some leafy greens, like spinach, Swiss chard, collard greens, parsley, leeks, and beet greens; berries; almonds; cashews; peanuts; soybeans; okra; quinoa; cocoa; tea; and chocolate. Oxalates may inhibit some of the absorption of calcium (and other minerals), but some may still be absorbed. Mixing up and varying the types of foods eaten on a regular basis encourages adequate absorption.
- Vitamin D levels. Serum levels of vitamin D need to be in optimum range in order to absorb calcium.
- High intakes of sodium, protein, caffeine, and phosphorus (from sodas) may enhance excretion of calcium.

The previous understanding of protein's effect on calcium was because it increased excretion of calcium, it contributed to loss of bone minerals. However, more recent evidence suggests that high protein intake also increases absorption of calcium by the intestines, thereby compensating for any losses.[11]

The bottom line is that we can maximize our intake of calcium-rich foods by spreading these foods throughout the day, enjoying them in different ways (raw, cooked, blended, intact, alone, in combination with other foods), and exercising consistently to promote healthy bone density.

Iodine

A trace element required in small quantities, iodine[12] is essential for life as a component of two thyroid hormones. These thyroid hormones control metabolism, protein synthesis, enzymatic activity, growth, development, and reproductive function. These hormones are also responsible for appropriate development in fetuses and infants, impacting skeletal and neurological maturity. Thyroid hormones are also essential in relation to your metabolism. Both a lack of adequate iodine intake and excessive intakes of iodine can lead to a goiter—or enlarged thyroid—an outwardly evident sign of thyroid dysfunction.

Iodine insufficiency is considered to be the world's most common cause of preventable brain damage. Disorders due to iodine deficiency span several different manifestations, including mental retardation, hypothyroidism, goiter, fatigue, weight gain, and cretinism.

At least two nutrients that may interact with iodine to exacerbate deficiency are selenium and goitrogens. A deficiency in selenium can worsen the consequences of iodine deficiency. Goitrogens are antinutrients found in cruciferous vegetables, soy products, flaxseeds, millet, peaches, pears, peanuts, pine nuts, spinach, sweet potatoes, and strawberries. If you have an iodine deficiency, these foods can disrupt your thyroid function. However, avoiding these healthy foods is unnecessary as long as your iodine intake is sufficient.

Dietary sources are unreliable and vary geographically. Essentially, iodine is best found in the oceans and in some soil found in certain areas around the world, dependent upon the location, fertilizer use, and irrigation practices. Sea vegetables—such as dulse and nori—are good sources for iodine.

Avoid hijiki seaweed (also spelled like hiziki) because it tends to be high in arsenic.

VEGI-SIDE

Small doses of iodized table salt are another way to increase your iodine intake. Each gram (1/4 to 1/8 teaspoon) of iodized salt in the United States should provide approximately 45 micrograms of iodine, meaning that it takes only about one-half teaspoon of iodized salt to provide the daily 150-microgram requirement. Note that most gourmet salts and salts found in processed foods, soy sauce, tamari, and miso are not iodized.

Iodine supplements are also available if sea vegetables or iodized salt is not an option.

Iron

Although iron is one of the most abundant metals on the planet, it is the most common and widespread nutritional deficiency in the world! It is also the only nutrient deficiency that is present significantly in industrial countries. It is especially prevalent in women of childbearing age, pregnant women, infants, children, teenage girls, as well as in anyone experiencing bleeding, such as people with ulcers, inflamed intestines due to malabsorptive disorders, or heavy menstruation.

Iron plays a key role in oxygen transport and storage throughout the body. It also functions as an essential component of hundreds of proteins and enzymes and is involved in energy metabolism, DNA synthesis, and cell growth and differentiation.

The recommended increase in iron intake for vegans is 1.8 times the RDA. Fortunately, this is easy to do with the wide presence of iron-rich food choices. Yet again, leafy greens and legumes score huge in this category, so including these foods often is advantageous. Other choices include soy products, dark chocolate (yum!), blackstrap molasses, tahini, pumpkin seeds, sunflower seeds, raisins, prunes, and cashews.

Absorption may be impaired with the intake of phytates, tannic acids from tea, calcium in dairy, fiber, polyphenols in coffee and cocoa, and certain spices (like turmeric, coriander, chilies, and tamarind). Avoiding this is as simple as eating iron-rich foods separately from these nutrients as much as possible. For example, drink your coffee or tea separate from your meals and mix up the combinations of your meals. One of the best tips for optimizing iron absorption is to eat iron-rich foods together with vitamin C-rich foods because the citric acid improves the solubility and helps the iron be better absorbed. Food combinations that illustrate this idea include: a green smoothie with leafy greens (iron) and fruit (vitamin C); salad greens (iron) with tomatoes and bell peppers (vitamin C); or bean chili (iron) using tomato sauce (vitamin C).

Magnesium

Magnesium is abundant in the body and the food supply. Stored primarily in our bones and muscles, magnesium is a cofactor in hundreds of enzyme systems, contributing to energy production and the synthesis of bone, nucleic acids (DNA and RNA), and protein. Also involved in transmitting nerve impulses, contracting muscles, and maintaining heart rhythm, magnesium is under tight regulation in the bloodstream, like calcium.

> **Magnesium—along with potassium, sodium, calcium, phosphate, chloride, and bicarbonate—is an electrolyte; along with other tasks, it helps regulate fluid balance in the body. Electrolytes are lost with excessive water loss, as during athletic activity, diarrhea, or vomiting, and need to be replaced via the diet to maintain homeostasis.**

VEGI-SIDE

As the RDA fluctuates throughout the lifespan, more details can be found in the charts beginning on page 243. Healthy sources of magnesium include leafy green vegetables (as usual), legumes (of course), nuts, peanuts and peanut butter, avocados, potatoes, bananas, apples, raisins, carrots, and whole grains. Magnesium is also a common ingredient in many medications, like laxatives and indigestion remedies.

Potassium

Another essential mineral and electrolyte, potassium is life-sustaining due to its role in regulating nerve impulse transmission, heart function, and muscle contraction. Potassium helps maintain fluid volume inside and outside of cells, contributing to cellular function. Hypokalemia, or low potassium, can occur with excessive fluid losses (fever, vomiting, diarrhea), the use of diuretics, some types of kidney disease, or heavy exercise without replenishment and is an imminent health concern as it can cause cardiac arrhythmias or muscle paralysis. Consuming a consistently adequate intake of potassium-rich foods, found mostly in fruits and vegetables, may help reduce risk for high blood pressure, bone loss, and kidney stones. Exceptional food sources include beet greens, lima beans, sweet potatoes, potatoes, spinach, and lentils.

Selenium

Like vitamins A, C, and E, selenium is a powerful antioxidant that protects the body against free radicals. This trace mineral is also important for multiple metabolic functions including the regulation of thyroid hormones, reproduction, and DNA synthesis. Selenium can be found in the soil, depending on the quality, and is stored in humans and animals primarily in muscle tissue. Just one ounce of Brazil nuts (which is a mere six to eight nuts) provides 777 percent of the RDA for selenium so one serving a week will provide all that we need. It can also be found in smaller, but healthy doses in whole grains, legumes, seeds, and other nuts.

Sodium

Perhaps the one micronutrient of which we are trying to eat *less*, sodium is an essential mineral and electrolyte necessary for life-sustaining processes like fluid balance, blood pressure, and nerve transmission.[13] We lose sodium naturally through perspiration, tears, and urine, but nutrient deficiency of sodium is rare. In acute situations, as in prolonged endurance exercise, hyponatremia—low blood sodium—is a life-threatening problem that can be fatal. This can also happen with excessive water intake or extreme fluid loss due to vomiting, diarrhea, diuretic use, and/or massive sweating. In all of these situations, electrolyte beverages may prevent or resolve the problem, but sometimes, medical attention is warranted.

On the flip side, many people overconsume sodium due to its ubiquitous presence in processed foods, fast foods, and restaurant meals. In fact, many people consume more than two times the adequate intake levels recommended. Chronically high intakes of sodium may promote high blood pressure and kidney problems in populations at high risk, like those with hypertension, diabetes, and kidney disease, as well as those who are over the age of 51 and/or are African American. For these populations, managing sodium intake is necessary. We only need approximately 180 to 500 milligrams a day to function, but the adequate intake level is set at 1,500 milligrams with an upper limit of less than 2,300 milligrams a day. Average consumption in the U.S. is 3,436 milligrams a day![14] Sodium is widely available in healthy doses in whole plant foods.

Zinc

Zinc is an essential trace mineral, supporting immune function and wound healing, synthesizing protein and DNA, and assisting growth and development throughout pregnancy, childhood, and adolescence.[15]

Although zinc status is difficult to measure using blood tests, clinical deficiency typically shows up as delayed wound healing, growth retardation, suppressed appetite, decreased immune function, hair loss, taste abnormalities, or eye and skin lesions. Those at risk include alcoholics and people consuming inadequate calories. Zinc deficiency may also exhibit in the presence of digestive diseases.

Daily intake is necessary and plant sources high in zinc are legumes, cashews and other nuts, seeds, soy products, and whole grains. Because of the concern of phytates disrupting absorption of zinc, it is recommended that people on a plant-based diet aim for 50 percent greater than the RDA intake of zinc. Similar to iron and calcium, methods like soaking, sprouting, leavening, and fermenting will reduce this effect and improve absorption.

The Real Deal about Supplements

Supplements are a dime a dozen these days; whether it's a big chain pharmacy or your local health food store, you're sure to see shelves and shelves of supplements. And the debate about their efficacy is only growing. Supplemental nutrients were initially intended to replete a deficiency—in which case, they can be effective. However, what has evolved is the idea that popping a pill filled with necessary or additional nutrients can compensate for a poor diet and keep us healthy—a nutritional "magic bullet." Not only is this a false notion, but this belief can be dangerous, harmful for several reasons.

First, to put it bluntly: a poor diet cannot be overcome by any pill or enough exercise. There is absolutely no substitute for a diet built on crucial, life-saving phytochemicals, fibers, vitamins, minerals, and antioxidants from real whole food sources. Proper nutrition is intrinsically, inherently the key to optimal wellness and to enabling the body to do its job by minimizing toxins and maximizing protection from unavoidable exposure to disease-promoting elements. On average, humans develop one cancer cell a day. We are also bombarded by viruses, bacteria, molds, fungi, radiation, free radicals, and other stressors that challenge our immune function every day. That is simply the world we live in. The only way to stay healthy is to maintain the integrity of the immune system— not to add stress—and we can do that consistently with the food we eat. Supplements do not come close to replicating this effect.

VEGI-SIDE

Probiotics are one category of supplements that have shown to have some potential health benefits. Because infinite types of beneficial bacteria are available, dosages range widely, and certain bacteria target different systems, choosing an appropriate formula is difficult. Always consult with your healthcare practitioner when deciding to utilize probiotics for more accurate recommendations.

Further, our bodies are not designed to take on concentrated doses of one nutrient in an isolated form. A recent study in the Annals of Internal Medicine[16] examined a very large database of supplement studies and concluded that certain supplements are harmful (specifically beta-carotene, vitamin E, and possibly high doses of vitamin A) while the others are ineffective for preventing illness and death due to chronic diseases. The headline of an accompanying editorial was "Enough Is Enough: Stop Wasting Money on Vitamin and Mineral Supplements."

Finally, and perhaps most alarming, the Dietary Supplement Health and Education Act (DSHEA) of 1994 legislated responsibility of safety directly to the supplement manufacturers. In other words, neither the federal government nor an objective third party is required to ensure the safety, efficacy, or consistency of products sold as supplements. In 2007, the FDA issued a set of requirements and expectations by which dietary supplements are manufactured, prepared, and stored to ensure quality, called Good Manufacturing Practices.[17] These practices suggest an expectation of the manufacturers to guarantee identity, purity, strength, and composition of their own products.

However, multiple studies performed time and time again on commercially sold products confirm that most supplements do not contain what their labels imply, contain sometimes dangerous additives not listed on the label, and/or do not contain the potency listed on the label. Warning letters are issued by the FDA when these discrepancies are caught, but it is likely impossible to maintain objective supervision over all the products on the market.

A few organizations—like Consumer Lab, NSF International, and U.S. Pharmacopeia—serve as independent third parties offering a stamp of approval after quality testing products for potency and contaminants. However, they do not confirm safety or efficacy. You can find these organizations online.

VEGI-SIDE

Ultimately, it is buyer beware. Because people eating a plant-based diet require vitamin B12 supplements, my recommendation is for a microalgae omega-3 source, and because vitamin D supplementation is necessary for many different people, my recommendation is to buy different brands when replenishing. Alternating products produced by different companies may minimize exposure to possible contaminants and maximize augmentation closest to desired potency. Healthcare providers can suggest brands they trust to provide safe and effective dietary supplements. For all other nutrients, focus on whole foods.

The Vegiterranean Diet for All

The nutrition recommendations in this chapter and throughout the book are geared toward the general adult population. Although the same nutrition instructions apply across the lifespan—as this is the most health-promoting way of eating for everyone—a few details are specific to pregnant women, infants, children, seniors, and athletes. If you've been diagnosed with a chronic illness or disease, are taking medications, or have allergies, you may require certain adjustments as well. For example, if you've been diagnosed with Celiac disease or have a gluten intolerance, you'll need to avoid gluten; some medications interact with foods (like vitamin K and blood-thinning medications).

If you have any questions about diet, you should always see a licensed healthcare practitioner. Preferably, look for a physician or registered dietitian who is well versed in a plant-based diet. Growing databases help to connect such experts to people.

Here are just a few notes about people who may have particular needs when making any dietary changes. My book *The Complete Idiot's Guide to Plant-Based Nutrition* provides more detailed information, as do the resources listed on pages 241–242.

Pregnant Women

Not only is pregnancy a special time emotionally, but it is perhaps the most important time in a woman's life to care for herself physically, as she becomes a temporary home for another being. Amazing and brilliant as that is, it comes with a few responsibilities. Throughout the physiological fluctuations of the approximately 40-week period, moms-to-be must remember to eat as nutritionally-dense as possible while avoiding toxins such as caffeine, alcohol, nicotine, artificial sweeteners, nitrites, fish, raw dairy, raw eggs, soft cheeses, as many additives as possible, and unsupervised medications, herbs, and supplements. The emphasis should be on wholesome, recognizable foods with as much color as possible.

Mindfulness is applicable in gauging how much to eat, and eating as healthfully as possible when you're hungry allows for the natural growth of your changing body. The first trimester is often exceptionally challenging in this regard, as nausea and fatigue make it difficult to eat certain healthful foods or even to go about preparing or buying them.

In these situations:

- Practicing self-compassion, knowing what's best for you, is all anyone can ask, and helps while riding these waves.
- A prenatal vitamin can act as insurance during rough patches, so talk with your healthcare provider about taking one a day during periods of time when nausea or exhaustion prevents you from eating plenty of nutrient-dense foods.
- If nothing sounds appealing, try whole-grain plain crackers, rice cakes, or brown rice.
- Ginger, found in tea, candy, and real ginger soda, is a natural remedy for nausea.
- Try small meals, or even just bites and sips, throughout the day— they do add up!
- Staying well hydrated is essential. When vomiting, an electrolyte beverage like coconut water can help you to replenish lost electrolytes.

Nutrient know-how during pregnancy very much relies on the same principles of the Vegiterranean Diet. No matter how you eat, iron-deficiency is common during pregnancy, because of the increased demand of iron for the fetus. Expectant moms should eat foods high in iron like leafy greens and beans as regularly as possible and eat them together with vitamin C-rich foods like citrus, strawberries, and tomatoes (nutrient synergy details are found in Chapter 2). Folate-rich foods (leafy greens and legumes) are also critical during pregnancy, as are sources of omega-3 fatty acids such as hemp, chia, or flaxseeds; walnuts; organic (or non-GMO specified) soy products; and leafy greens. Pregnant women who are not adamant about omega-3-rich foods may benefit from supplementing with microalgae DHA during pregnancy, as well as throughout lactation. An exercise routine can be continued with mild modification, as necessary. A vitamin B12 supplement is as indispensable as always. Most pressing? Resting as much as possible.

Breastfeeding Moms

For the first few weeks, an infant's sole source of nutrition comes from breast milk or, if not possible, formula. Whatever a breastfeeding mom eats, the baby eats. This is when making every bite count matters more than ever (no pressure, right?). Highly nutritious foods such as leafy greens, legumes, nuts, and seeds infuse nutrition into breast milk. Breast milk is the most nutrient-dense food for an infant, providing a baby with the baseline for his or her immune system and nourishment to sustain the incredibly rapid growth that occurs in those first few months.

Breastfeeding can sustain your baby for the first six months alone, after which other foods are added to supplement and then ultimately replace the milk.

Lactation requires the same nutritional pattern of eating as pregnancy, except sustaining milk production calls for more calories. Hydration is still crucial. To echo pregnancy rhetoric, a vitamin B12 supplement is as indispensable as ever. Plus, breastfeeding moms who are not adamant about eating omega-3-rich foods should consider supplementing with microalgae DHA, as it is vital for your baby's brain development.

VEGI-SIDE

During pregnancy and lactation, nutrient requirements are increased in most categories so checking the DRI tables is helpful.

Infants

Infants rely on liquid exclusively until about six months of age. If breastfeeding is not an option, a commercial infant formula should be substituted. As of now, the choice is between a soy or dairy formula. Because of the potential association between early dairy consumption and type 1 diabetes[18,19] and allergies,[20] soy may be the better alternative. After six months, the exciting progression of learning how to eat begins (this process may last an entire lifetime, really)! Introducing solids to your baby is a tedious, yet fascinating process. Iron-fortified cereals begin your little one's gastronomical journey, typically rice being first. Precise execution in timing, allowing a few days in between new food introductions, will help you monitor for potential allergies. Following cereals, you can slowly add pureed vegetables and fruits, one at a time. Then, you can bulk up calorie intake with foods like mashed avocados, tofu, beans, and lentils; nut and seed butters; plant yogurts; and pureed soups.

At around four to six months of age, your baby's stored iron levels (collected while in utero) start running out. This is why infant cereals are formulated with iron. Moms who choose to make their own cereals need to provide sources of supplemental iron from other foods or dietary supplements that meet the requirements for babies, which is eleven milligrams a day from age seven to twelve months. Infants on formula can typically meet iron needs. Your pediatrician can answer any questions, offering suggestions and guidelines.

Once your baby shows signs that he is ready to eat chunkier, more textured foods, items should be introduced very slowly. A good start is by making any purees less smooth, or cut avocado and tofu chunks slightly larger and larger. Somewhere between nine and eleven months, your baby may seem interested in trying more grown-up finger foods. Again, to avoid choking potential, you'll want to initiate soft items slowly; foods such as pastas, breads, peas, lentils, beans, tofu, potatoes, yams, bananas, and other soft fruits like ripe mango and papaya, and steamed vegetables are good choices.

As your baby progresses, he can begin eating unsweetened cereals, tortillas, crackers, teething biscuits, lightly cooked vegetables, tempeh, and some of the foods your family enjoys together. Following your baby's lead, while closely monitoring his progress, leads to a safe and organic experience.

VEGI-SIDE

Children

As a mom of two, I know quite well how challenging it is not only to encourage kids to eat healthfully, but to be constantly inundated by saboteurs in the classroom, at parties, at sports practices and games, around relatives and friends, and essentially anywhere outside of the home (commonly even within the home). Sometimes it feels like a war between knowing what is right in feeding your kids and the concern of psychologically scarring them by constantly saying no to the incessant offering of junk. What is a health-conscientious parent to do? Here are some of the most effective actions for proactively setting up your off-spring for a lifetime of health:

- Meals prepared at home supply the best nutrition. Packing any snacks, lunches, or other meals for on-the-go and always having something safe on standby can thwart saboteurs.
- When dining out, children's menus should be avoided since the choices are almost always nutritionally void. A more nutritious adult meal may be split between your children, shared with an adult, or enjoyed then and again later as leftovers. A healthier appetizer may be another option.
- Role-modeling is the number one most important influence on a child's future eating patterns. "Do as I say *as well* as what I do" is a healthy credo to really live every day when it comes to good food.
- Health-promoting foods must always be available and easily visible. If your kitchen is stocked with brightly colored, ready-to-eat, delicious treats, chances are that is what your child will automatically grab.
- Keep it fun and engaging. The more involved your children are in meal planning and preparation, the more they will feel invested in the end product and will want to enjoy it.

Nutritionally speaking, children can follow the principles of the Vegiterranean Diet, only cutting down the proportions. In other words, the same foods and same portion ratios can be used, but the amount of servings are decreased to meet a child's caloric requirements. Her plate should still be half filled with fruits and vegetables, with legumes, whole grains, and nuts and seeds rounding out the remainder. You should also encourage your child to honor her hunger/satiety levels. Allowing your child not to eat when she is not hungry—even if it is time for a meal—and not forcing her to finish a meal when she is full will develop and hone these essential intuitive skills for life.

Age-specific nutrient needs are detailed in "Nutrient Charts and Tables" beginning on page 243. As discussed earlier in this chapter, a child should ideally also take a B12 supplement. A pediatrician should monitor vitamin D levels with recommended blood work. If a deficiency is detected, safe sunshine exposure, D-fortified plant milks and cereals, and supplements can be considered. A regular source of iodine, via one-quarter teaspoon of iodized salt or even a periodic multivitamin, is also strongly recommended. Talk with your pediatrician about multivitamin supplementation.

Seniors

Typical aging brings about physiological changes that may present new nutritional challenges such as losing skeletal muscle and increasing fat, a decreasing ability to digest and absorb nutrients, decreased appetite, chewing difficulties, mobility limitations, and side effects of medications. Unfortunately as a result, malnutrition is all too common.

But aging unto itself doesn't have to be problematic, especially if you've had a healthy diet and sustained regular physical activity. Plant-based eaters tend to live longer and maintain their vitality well into their older years, avoiding common multiple medications and maintaining agility. After age sixty-five, it is time to take a blatant, objective look at how you are moving and what you are eating. Resistance exercise and weight-bearing cardiovascular exercise like walking can manage muscles and bones. Balance and coordination exercises are also critical to avoid frailty. Since metabolism slows with age, keeping tabs on your body weight can help you avoid chronic diseases. Eating should be a conscious undertaking to sustain your health.

If you're over sixty-five, you should be more aware of the following nutrients: fiber, protein, calcium, iron, and vitamins B6, B12, and D. Since many seniors have a sluggish digestive system, adequate hydration is especially important. To get more liquids into your diet without feeling like you have to drink gallons and gallons, your diet can include soups, smoothies, and plenty of roughage from fruits and vegetables.

Protein intakes are often low in seniors, regardless of their dietary patterns. Although it is healthful to eat lower amounts of protein in younger adult life, after age sixty-five, levels of IGF-1 decrease and it becomes safer to consume a more sizable intake of protein. Ways to amp up your protein include eating more bean-based foods, soy products, an ounce of nuts a day, nut and seed butters, leafy greens, and even a whole food plant protein powder may help.

VEGI-SIDE

For an in-depth exploration of the world's longest-lived populations and a huge dose of inspiration, I highly recommend the book, *The Blue Zones*.[21]

Optimal levels of vitamin D and adequate intake of calcium-rich foods support bone health. Seniors need a B12 supplement of 500 to 1,000 micrograms daily, as discussed earlier. Iron-deficiency is common, but usually due to factors other than a senior's diet. To reduce risk for anemia, seniors should be especially attuned to food combining with vitamin C- and iron-rich foods. At least four servings of fruit a day plus beans, avocados, leafy greens, nuts, and seeds supplies the necessary amounts of vitamin B6.

Ultimately, eating a whole food, plant-based Vegiterranean diet sets up a senior for success. And it is truly never too late to start.

Athletes

Taking the body to heightened levels of exertion requires optimal nutrients for both performance and recovery. Plant-strong athletes have been taking the world by storm with exceptional results, and the appeal and popularity of this diet is continuously growing. Out of the multitude of benefits of eating a diet loaded with phytochemicals and antioxidants, superior recovery is the cornerstone. With accelerated recovery comes more efficient training and, therefore, optimized performance. Prolonged or intense exercise inherently promotes muscle breakdown and oxidation, essentially invoking an internal microscopic onslaught. Flooding the body's system with nutrients that initiate repair, recovery, and rejuvenation helps bring about positive adaptation and enables reaching the next level of training more rapidly.

Nutrient-dense Vegiterranean meals can be planned around training. The most important meal of the day is the immediate post-recovery meal. Within 30 to 45 minutes after a workout, your body is most ready, willing, and able to absorb nutrients. This is the time to replenish your glycogen stores and quench free radicals brought on during a workout. For rapid digestion and absorption into the body, your focus should be on foods rich in simple carbohydrates, lower in fat, and lower in protein, which also help to speed glycogen synthesis. Plenty of antioxidants from colorful fruits and/or vegetables will help quench free radicals.

Hydration is crucial in all types of fitness but it is especially critical if you are endurance training. Staying well hydrated protects your body from potentially fatal risks related to dehydration. Drinking water alone will suffice for up to 60 to 90 minutes of consistent activity. After that, your body begins to lose electrolytes, which need to be replenished to avoid hyponatremia, an abnormally low blood level of sodium which causes cells to malfunction and can be fatal. See page 190 for a delicious, natural sports drink recipe that will help sustain you during endurance activities.

Carbohydrates are an athlete's best tool, as they fuel exercise immediately and over an extended period of time via energy storage (glycogen). Simple carbs from fruits (fresh and dried) and green smoothies eaten immediately before a workout or event are quickly absorbed into the bloodstream, providing immediate fuel. To build up glycogen storage slowly, more complex carbs from whole grains, starchy vegetables, and legumes can be included during the rest of the day.

Protein requirements for endurance and strength-trained athletes are slightly higher than the IOM RDA.[22] Recommendations are set at a range 1.2 to 1.7 grams per kilogram bodyweight per day. If you're an athlete, the vegiterranean diet can help you maximize both your performance and recovery.

Weight Loss

Losing weight is a topic that's never simple, regardless of your situation. Weight loss is additionally complex in the way that our food supply has shifted, hormones and toxins have contributed to excess weight, and society has made it extraordinarily challenging to eat only enough to maintain a healthy body weight.

A large part of the problem is the hyper-accessibility of hyper-palatable food. The best solution is to avoid these foods altogether, so as to break the addictive cycle, at least for a while, until the taste buds have recalibrated. Eating whole plant foods and omitting processed and animal products is the best way to achieve results because plant foods are naturally low in calories, high in satisfying fiber, and high in nutrition to balance out your body chemistry.

The Vegiterranean Diet is built to break away from the hyper-palatable food addictions and reset your hormones and taste buds to eat the right foods for weight loss—and healthy weight maintenance. It's also important to remember to treat yourself in a compassionate, holistic manner. Cautious Calorie Consciousness (CCC, as discussed in Chapter 4) and mindfulness when directly focusing on food are especially helpful when your goal is weight loss. In addition, the emotional component must be addressed.

Food journals logging emotions and hunger/satiety levels monitor what works and does not work and may expose your triggers to overeating. Go-to lists of activities to swap out for eating when we are stressed, tired, anxious, or depressed (or experiencing any other emotion we quell with food) can save you at the moment of weakness. With this information in hand, you can also pick treats that excite you, such as reading a good magazine or book for pure pleasure, taking a long, hot bath, calling a friend, spending quality time with a pet, or watching a fun movie or television show. Go-to lists of beloved activities allow you to practice asking yourself if you are truly hungry before you eat. If you find yourself reaching for a snack because of any reason other than hunger, grab your list and commit to one of those other non-food activities. Changing course and addressing your body's and mind's real needs lead to relaxation, fun, or connection.

If you feel like you're really in a rut with emotional eating, you may want consider professional assistance. So many different types of therapy are incredibly effective and provide support as you focus on our health from the inside out, offering tools to help navigate through the journey.

Support can come from friends and family as well. A support network is crucial for emotional wellbeing. You can make connections with people facing similar experiences through online groups, in social media, and from local in-person meet ups. Being healthy literally takes a village, but that is precisely what the village is for ... to help sustain its people. Weight loss is absolutely doable and sustainable for anyone, so long as you approach it from all of these different angles, addressing the ones that impact you the most, and remaining gentle with yourself throughout the process. If you're not sure where to start, the Resources on pages 241–242 offer help.

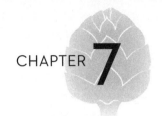
Stile di Vita...

Strategies, Meal Plans, and Navigating the World

As a busy, working, full-time mama, I like making meal preparation as simple as possible. Thus, I am a huge fan of one-pot wonders, one weekly prep day, batch cooking, and staying flexible. To make things even more challenging (entertaining?) in my home, I have two picky kids and an even pickier husband, all preferring and despising different foods, I might add. So, I tend to focus on buffet-style eating, side dishes, and plenty of variety, which also happens to be classic Mediterranean style, anyway. For those who have a less complicated situation, meeting needs may be simpler—and suggestions found here may be easily adjusted accordingly.

Buffet-style eating is an efficient method of serving food by having multiple options spread out and enabling diners to serve themselves. Despite its traditional commonality around the globe, a buffet spread is only recently increasing in popularity in the United States. It is a wonderful way to incorporate variety and to ensure plenty of leftovers.

VEGI-SIDE

Because life is unpredictable and eating healthfully requires some level of preparation, I designed the Vegiterranean Meal Plan to be flexible and customizable for you and your family. Instead of creating a rigid guide, I

In this chapter you'll learn...
- *Strategies for success: the ACHIEVE method and the Five Tools to help you goal-plan and minimize stress.*
- *Twenty-one days of meals plus suggestions for easy menu planning.*
- *Tips for dining out, visiting friends and family, and traveling a la Vegiterranean.*

am offering a variety of options for breakfasts, lunches, dinners, snacks, and even desserts. This way, if you prefer enjoying last night's dinner leftovers for lunch the next day you won't feel as if you've taken a big detour from the plan. Or, if like me, you prefer eating a little bit of a lot of different foods at one meal, you can happily do so. Eating healthy should be easy and adaptable to your own schedule, rather than strict, stressful, and difficult. Even more importantly, this format lends itself to an important theme of the Vegiterranean diet—listening to your inner signals and practicing mindfulness. Not only should eating be nutritious, it should be pleasurable and practical, especially to keep it simple and sustainable.

If we analyzed how many meals we rely on per week, the average person shuffles between one to three different breakfasts, two to four lunches, and three to five dinners. Many people eat the same thing every day! Consistency is priceless and setting out a regular routine is realistic. As mentioned throughout this book, no single diet formula is perfect, no secret number for how many meals and/or snacks is ideal, and no exact sequence of eating is right for everyone. What is "perfect" is holding onto some basic, critical principles, and then maneuvering them to work for each one of us. This community-oriented way of eating lends itself to a very individualized eating plan.

VEGI-SIDE

Although constancy is common and comforting, variety literally is the spice of life and key to maximizing nutrition. A happy compromise is to switch up the little things within our comfort parameters, such as alternating the type of leafy greens we put in a salad, the type of plant milk we use in our oatmeal, and the beans we choose to make hummus. This ensures an overall broader intake of nutrients.

Five Tips for Easy Meal Planning

If you are new to eating plant-based, here are five tips for navigating meal planning with ease:

1. Start with the foods and types of recipes that you love. If it appeals to you, excites you, inspires you, focus on those. If you hate celery but

fantasize about kale, don't force yourself to eat celery. Eat more kale, instead. If you love meatloaf, test out plant-based versions made with lentils, beans, and/or mushrooms until you find one that you crave. There is no lack in the plant kingdom and the arsenal of possible options is infinite.

2. Focus on variety. As I mentioned earlier, most of us get stuck in a rut of rotating through just a short list of foods. Yet, it is advantageous to leave the comfort zone a bit here and there and expand our horizons by testing out new foods. Experiment with seasonal and local produce, different varieties of whole grains or legumes, and substituting alternate ingredients in recipes, such as almond milk instead of rice milk or quinoa instead of brown rice to keep shaking things up.

3. If you have a craving, distract before delving. First rule of thumb is to determine if you are truly hungry, as discussed in Chapter 4. When it is psychological and you do not feel physical hunger, employ your list of favorite pleasurable (non-eating) activities. If you are actually hungry and craving something sweet, try a piece of fruit, a green juice, a green smoothie, blended frozen fruit, a serving of sweet vegetables, such as sweet potatoes, yams, carrots, or beets, or any of the sweet recipes in this book. If it is something salty you are craving, try sea vegetables, nutritional yeast, a savory recipe from Chapter 9, or something sour, like citrus, to distract your taste buds. On the other hand, if there is a recipe you used to enjoy, try swapping out the animal and/or processed ingredients with whole plant options. Examples of healthy swaps are peppered throughout Chapter 8.

4. Aim for leftovers. Plan ahead by selecting the meals you (and your family) will be consuming ahead of time, shopping with lists, and preparing adequate amounts of food. Think ahead by making extras for the next day or two, or even to freeze for the near future. Knowing there are delicious options in plentitude in your kitchen provides peace and pleasure, helping keep you on track and satisfied.

5. Mix and match. Forget following the meal plan precisely because it is a magic formula to success. Instead, use the meal plan as a guide for ideas on meal choices. For example, I happen to prefer vegetables for breakfast. Although that may sound a bit odd, I choose to eat vegetables

for breakfast, anyway. If you like dinner for breakfast or breakfast for dinner, my hat is off to you and you have my blessings! No judgment. No pressure. Simply personalized for your liking.

Meal Suggestions and Plans

Since they say it takes approximately twenty-one days to change your taste buds, here are twenty-one days worth of meals, a plethora of Vegiterranean-style choices for breakfasts, lunches, dinners, snacks, and desserts to mix and match according to preferences. Those suggestions marked with a star (*) are recipes found in Chapter 9. The rules are there are no rules. Simply listening to our bodies will guide portions and allow us to savor each meal.

BREAKFAST CHOICES:

1. Brain-Boosting Blue Smoothie*

2. Pumpkin Pie Green Smoothie*

3. Chocolate banana smoothie: 2 cups leafy greens, 1 medium frozen banana, 1/2 cup frozen blueberries, 2 cups unsweetened chocolate plant milk, 2 tablespoons nut butter (optional), 2 to 3 pitted dates (optional)

4. Fresh-pressed green juice with cucumbers; greens such as kale, dandelion greens, collard greens; carrots; beets; and a bit of fruit, such as pineapple, apple, or citrus

5. Moroccan Mint Chia Tea*

6. Oatmeal: plain or with plant milk, fruit (fresh or frozen), optional seeds, and/or nuts

7. *Quinoa Belila* (Traditional Egyptian Hot Cereal)*

8. *Shakshuka* (Middle Eastern Tofu Scramble)*

9. Breakfast Sunshine Salad*

10. Carrot Muffins*

11. Unsweetened whole-grain (rice, corn, wheat, oat) cold cereal with plant milk, seeds, and/or fruit

12. Baked beans in a bowl or on whole grain toast with fresh tomato slices

13. Banana Sandwich*

14. Baked Oat Bread,* toasted, with whole-fruit jam, apple butter, nut or seed butter, hummus, or mashed avocado

15. Plant-based yogurt with fresh fruit and a small handful of nuts or tablespoon of seeds

16. Scrambled tofu in vegetable broth with vegetables and spices, such as turmeric to make it yellow (and add flavor and nutrition) and pepper, plus nutritional yeast (optional), served with whole grain pita or wrapped in a whole grain tortilla

17. Baked sweet potato or yam drizzled with a teaspoon of pure maple syrup and sprinkled with cinnamon

18. Corn thins, rice cakes, or (sprouted) whole grain toast with thin layers of tofu or mashed avocado and thinly sliced tomatoes

19. Steamed leafy greens with a splash of fresh lemon juice, (balsamic) vinegar, or an oil-free dressing (choose from those in Chapter 9)

20. Brown rice pudding: cooked brown rice simmered in plant milk with cinnamon, vanilla extract, and a bit of pure maple syrup

21. Blueberry banana pancakes: mashed medium banana with 1/4 cup plant milk, 1 cup whole grain flour, 2 teaspoons baking powder, a tablespoon pure maple syrup, and a cup of fresh or thawed frozen blueberries, combined, divided, and cooked on the stovetop in a pan or skillet until golden brown

LUNCH CHOICES:

1. Vegiterranean Wrap: whole-grain tortilla, Hummus of the Earth*, thinly sliced bell peppers, cucumbers, soaked sun-dried tomatoes, romaine lettuce, and/or sprouts

2. Large salad with fresh greens, beans, shredded carrots, shredded beets, broccoli florets, and Lemon Basil Dressing*

3. Classic Caesar Salad: romaine lettuce, whole-grain croutons, Betta' than Feta*, Cashew Caesar Dressing*

4. Tuscan Garden Salad with Fresh Tomato Dressing*

5. Arugula salad with shaved fennel, white beans, and Peach Champagne Vinaigrette*

6. Baked Oat Bread* with Almond Sun-Dried Tomato Hummus* and sliced cucumbers

7. Quinoa Chickpea Taboulleh Salad*

8. Potato Corn Chowder*

9. Vegetable soup with beans and a whole grain roll

10. Sandwich on whole grain bread, spread avocado or hummus, and veggies

11. *Hatz* Lentil Soup* and Baked Oat Bread*

12. Tempeh Cutlet Sandwich with Arugula, and Basil Aioli*

13. Baked potato with beans, corn, steamed broccoli and salsa or oil-free dressing

14. Whole grain pita bread spread with hummus or Baba Ganoush* and stuffed with Israeli Salad*, sprouts and/or leafy greens

15. Roasted Vegetable Sandwich Rolls*

16. Soft tacos with whole grain tortillas, cooked lentils spiced with taco seasoning, shredded greens, fresh tomatoes, avocado or guacamole, and salsa

17. Potato Cups* or baked potato stuffed with Hearty Red Lentil Stew*

18. Noritos: in a nori wrapper (or whole grain tortilla), spread a thin layer of hummus, bean spread, miso paste, or guacamole, then add julienned vegetables, and wrap tightly

19. Veggie burger on whole grain bun with romaine lettuce, tomato slices, and baked potato wedges

20. Pizza with whole grain crust, marinara sauce, and loaded with veggies and Parma Shake*

21. *Ful Medames**

DINNER CHOICES:

1. Falafel* on pita or over salad with Tahina* and Israeli salad*

2. Veggie Pancakes* with dressing or hummus of choice and a side salad or cooked leafy greens

3. *Mujadara** with a side salad

4. Whole-grain pasta with cooked vegetables and *Sofrito** sauce or jarred oil-free marinara sauce and Parma Shake*

5. Cheesy Smoky Butternut Squash Pasta* with Roasted Vegetable Side Dish*

6. Red Hot Eggplant Salad* with whole-grain pita, Tahina*, and green salad

7. Green Ful* and whole grain pita, hummus or Baba Ganoush*, and Israeli Salad*

8. Hearty Red Lentil Stew* and Stone-ground Cornbread*

9. Easy Caprese* with whole grain bread

10. Vegiterranean plate with Tabbouleh,* Israeli Salad,* hummus or Tahina,*and pita bread or baked potato

11. Hot, Sweet, and Sour *Bhamia* (Okra)* and a side salad

12. Couscous Soup*

13. Vegiterranean Bowl: choice of whole grains, choice of beans and/or lentils, salad, cooked veggies, topped with oil-free dressing and/or a dollop of hummus or Tahina*

14. Plate of Dips: a sampler of different bean dips, hummus, Baba Ganoush* with crudité (e.g. broccoli florets, bell pepper strips, carrot sticks, celery sticks, jicama) and toasted whole grain tortillas, bread, pita or baked potato wedges

15. Pasta Primavera in reverse: small amount of whole grain pasta loaded with veggies and tossed with balsamic vinegar, lemon juice, fresh herbs, Sofrito,* jarred oil-free marinara sauce, or oil-free dressing and Parma Shake*

16. Delicious Dolmas* with Red Hot Eggplant Salad*

17. Polenta with Mushroom Ragu* and Lemon Chard with Chickpeas*

18. Wild rice with lentils, accompanied by steamed greens and oil-free dressing

19. Moussaka* with Dilled Rice with Lima Beans*

20. Quinoa with chickpeas, steamed veggies, and oil-free dressing

21. Rainbow Stuffed Cabbage Rolls* with Green *Fassulia* (Green Beans) and Potatoes*

SNACKS:

- Air-popped popcorn sprinkled with nutritional yeast and optional spices (i.e., chili powder or Italian spices)
- Fresh-pressed green juice
- Fresh seasonal fruit
- Moroccan Mint Chia Tea*

- Sunrise Kale Chips*
- Hummus of the Earth* with crudité
- Easy Caprese*
- Baba Ganoush* with whole-grain crackers
- Smoky Avocado Dip* with toasted corn tortillas and salsa
- Potato Cups* stuffed with hummus, guacamole, and/or salsa
- White Bean and Rosemary Dip* with whole-grain crackers

DESSERTS:

- Almond-Stuffed Baked Apple Cups*
- Summer Fruit Tart*
- Frozen blended fruit, such as bananas with a sprinkle of cocoa powder
- Ganache Parfait with Poached Berries*
- Chocolate Hazelnut Chia Pudding*
- Grilled Nectarines with Amaretto Gelato*
- Italian Wedding Cookies*
- Chocolate Crispy Fruit Squares*

BEVERAGES:

- Water: ideally throughout the day and between meals (approximately half your weight in pounds in ounces of water per day on average)
- Coconut water can be enjoyed as a sports beverage or for a delicious treat (minding the fact that it is not replacing water due to the fact that it contains calories)
- Plant milks: opt for unsweetened and experiment with almond, soy, rice, hemp, and oat for use as a beverage, in recipes, and to replace dairy milk
- Tea: black, green, white, oolong, and herbal; hot and/or iced
- Coffee: decaf or regular (unless you are sensitive)
- Green juices: treat these as light meals instead of as a beverage to go alongside a meal
- Green smoothies: as with green juices, these are meals, not side beverages, and will keep you full for longer than a juice because of the retained fiber

CONDIMENTS:

- Mustards: all types, including Dijon, spicy brown, and yellow
- Vinegars: all types, especially apple cider, balsamic, rice, red wine
- Fresh and dried herbs and spices (see Chapter 8 for more details)
- Nutritional yeast
- Hot sauce
- Salsa

Up to two or three eight-ounce servings of caffeine each day is fine for the general population. If you have high blood pressure, irregular heart rhythms, anxiety, stress, sleep problems, ulcers, acid reflux, chronic headaches, or are pregnant, it is best to avoid caffeine or, at least, discuss with your physician for specific guidelines.

VEGI-SIDE

Sample Meal Plans

Now that you have twenty-one breakfast, lunch, dinner, and snack ideas, you can arrange them according to your tastes and schedule. Use this week of sample meal plans as a template for ideas on how a Vegiterranean day-in-the-life may look. As always, these are interchangeable so meals may be mixed up as desired, portions eaten to match hunger/satiety, and follow personal preferences.

Sample Meal Plan 1

BREAKFAST: Brain-Boosting Blue Smoothie*

SNACK (OPTIONAL): Hummus of the Earth* with raw baby carrots, celery sticks, and broccoli florets

LUNCH: Roasted Vegetable Sandwich Rolls*

DINNER: Cheesy Smoky Butternut Squash Pasta* with Roasted Vegetable Side Dish*

DESSERT (OPTIONAL): Chocolate Hazelnut Chia Pudding*

Sample Meal Plan 2

BREAKFAST: Oatmeal, plain or add plant milk, fruit (fresh or frozen), seeds, and/or nuts

SNACK (OPTIONAL): Fresh seasonal fruit

LUNCH: Classic Caesar Salad: romaine lettuce, whole grain croutons, Betta' than Feta,* Cashew Caesar Dressing*

DINNER: Hearty Red Lentil Stew* and Stone-ground Cornbread

DESSERT (OPTIONAL): Almond-Stuffed Baked Apple Cups*

Sample Meal Plan 3

BREAKFAST: Carrot Muffins*

SNACK (OPTIONAL): White Bean and Rosemary Dip* with whole-grain crackers

LUNCH: Potato Cups* stuffed with hummus, guacamole, and/or salsa

DINNER: *Mujadara** with side green salad

DESSERT (OPTIONAL): Chocolate Crispy Fruit Squares*

Sample Meal Plan 4

BREAKFAST: Pumpkin Pie Green Smoothie*

SNACK (OPTIONAL): Smoky Avocado Dip* with toasted corn tortillas and salsa

LUNCH: Tuscan Garden Salad with Fresh Tomato Dressing*

DINNER: Falafel* on pita with Tahina* and Israeli salad*

DESSERT (OPTIONAL): Italian Wedding Cookies*

Sample Meal Plan 5

BREAKFAST: Fresh-pressed green juice with cucumbers, kale, dandelion greens, collard greens, carrots, and/or seasonal fruit

SNACK (OPTIONAL): Easy Caprese*

LUNCH: Quinoa Chickpea Taboulleh Salad*

DINNER: Veggie Pancakes* with dressing or hummus of choice and a side salad or cooked leafy greens

DESSERT (OPTIONAL): Summer Fruit Tart*

Sample Meal Plan 6

BREAKFAST: Baked Oat Bread,* toasted, with whole-fruit jam

SNACK (OPTIONAL): Air-popped popcorn sprinkled with nutritional yeast and optional spices (i.e., chili powder or Italian spices)

LUNCH: Arugula salad with shaved fennel, white beans, and Peach Champagne Vinaigrette*

DINNER: Dolmas* with Couscous Soup*

DESSERT (OPTIONAL): Grilled Nectarines with Amaretto Gelato*

Sample Meal Plan 7

BREAKFAST: Breakfast Sunshine Salad*

SNACK (OPTIONAL): Moroccan Mint Chia Tea*

LUNCH: Tempeh Cutlet Sandwich with Arugula and Basil Aioli*

DINNER: Moussaka* and Dilled Rice with Lima Beans*

DESSERT (OPTIONAL): Ganache Parfait with Poached Berries*

Keeping It Simple

All of the meal plan and recipe suggestions are examples of ways to put together basic Vegiterranean foods. A simpler method that can be used overall, is to streamline further and have meals that are literally just a few plain foods. Here are some examples of a week of fabulously healthful, Vegiterranean plates that require very little preparation:

BREAKFASTS:

- An apple or banana with almond butter
- Lots of fresh berries or other fruits
- Smoothie of kale, berries, pineapple, and unsweetened almond milk
- Smoothie of spinach, mango, banana, and coconut water
- Cooked quinoa with a drizzle of maple syrup and shake of cinnamon
- A bowl of plain cooked oatmeal and a banana
- Whole-grain toast with nut butter, mashed avocado, apple butter

LUNCHES:

- Plain cooked quinoa, steamed kale, some cooked beans, and a dressing or hummus on top
- Salad with beans and oil-free dressing
- Baked potato with mustard and cooked broccoli
- Sandwich with whole-grain bread, hummus, and veggies
- Vegetable-based soup with whole-grain bread
- Soup and salad
- Burrito with whole-grain tortilla, rice, beans, avocado, veggies, and salsa

DINNERS:

- Cooked wild rice, beans, cooked veggies, oil-free dressing
- Veggie burger and baked potato wedges
- Whole-grain pasta with marinara sauce and vegetables
- Corn, beans, rice, with vegetables (salad and/or cooked)
- Lentils, rice, with vegetables (salad and/or cooked)
- Tofu or tempeh and vegetable stir-fry over brown rice
- Cheeseless pizza (store-bought crust or on pita bread, tortilla, or whole-grain bagel) with marinara sauce and loaded with veggies

Boom. Easy. Wholesome food. These ideas can frame a schedule, and then you can pepper in the recipes from Chapter 9 throughout the week whenever you have more time to cook. Cooking big batches and storing the leftovers means less prep time on subsequent days. The simpler, the better. Learning to prepare food for the first time or to prepare it differently than one is used to is like learning a new language. It starts with a few words—then, some phrases. Slowly, but steadily, the language becomes fluent and flowing. We can become fluent in whole food, plant-based Vegiterranean cooking with consistency.

KID-FRIENDLY MEAL IDEAS:

"Picky" and "kids" are typically two words glued together like peanut butter and jelly, so here are some options that are likely to smoothly wiggle their way onto a kid's plate:

- Whole-grain bagels with nut butters, jams, or hummus
- Pancakes or waffles with fresh fruit and pure maple syrup
- Tofu and veggie scramble
- Green smoothies
- Veggie burgers with baked potato wedges
- Bean burritos or tacos on whole grain tortillas or taco shells
- Nut or seed butter and whole fruit jam or banana sandwiches
- Pasta with marinara sauce
- DIY pizza with crust, marinara sauce, and favorite veggies and/or pineapple

Some great snacks for kids include:

- Trail mixes of nuts, seeds, dried or dehydrated fruits, and/or dark chocolate
- Whole food raw bars made from just dried fruits, nuts, seeds, nut butters, and/or dark chocolate
- Chia puddings
- Nut or seed butters spread on fruit
- Hummus or other (bean) dips with crackers or raw veggies
- Baked tortilla chips and salsa and/or guacamole
- Popcorn with nutritional yeast
- Ants on a log (celery sticks with nut butter and raisins) or banana boats (same thing but on bananas instead of celery)
- Fruit kabobs

POST-TRAINING MEAL EXAMPLES:

And for the athletes or exercise enthusiasts who burn through calories with gusto, here are some perfect post-workout meals to support recovery and overall training success:

- Green smoothie with leafy greens, fruits, and coconut water
- Whole grains (brown rice, quinoa, amaranth, buckwheat, wild rice) or corn with legumes (beans, lentils, or peas) and raw or cooked green (and other) vegetables (i.e., salad or steamed veggies)

- Burrito with whole-grain tortilla, filled with beans, rice, corn, and salsa with green salad
- Whole-grain pasta with oil-free marinara sauce
- Kale salad with beans, oil-free dressing, and whole-grain bread
- Baked (sweet) potato or yam with baked beans and broccoli or other vegetables

OUT AND ABOUT

Living Vegiterranean is not simply about following the Veg Ten and the Food Pyramid and achieving optimal nutrient status. As we saw in the Crete survey and the Seven Countries Study, there is more than meets the plate when it comes to living healthfully. Beyond nutritious food, movement, and mindfulness are motivation and maneuvering through the real world when dining out and traveling. Here are some successful navigation strategies.

MOTIVATION

You can lead a human to healthy, but you can't always make them eat! After working with hundreds of people over the years, I have found that regardless of how badly someone may want to change (become healthier, reduce stress, lose weight, etc.) or how knowledgeable he or she is about what needs to happen in order to do so, motivation is essential. Sure, people go on diets all the time and have great success losing weight. But the statistics[1] show that at least 80 to 90 percent of successful dieters gain all of the weight back (and sometimes more). Not only is this disappointing, but the physical and psychological consequences are counterproductive.

So how do we inspire ourselves (and others) to make positive, sustainable changes? Behavioral science has evolved over time, and some recent thinking helps solve this major dilemma. Recent evidence suggests that the most effective strategy is to focus on habits—creating health through simple habits.

A.C.H.I.E.V.E.

To help realize health goals by setting habits, it helps to first identify exactly what they are. You can focus by creating a list of bigger picture goals and dividing them into small habits. Use my A.C.H.I.E.V.E.—Affirmative Convenient Habitual Infinitesimal Effortless Victorious Exact—guideline:

Affirmative: Goals and habits need to be positive, optimistic, and happy. An example would be to replace "stop eating animal products" with "start eating more whole plant foods."

Convenient: Goals and habits should fit into the day where they most easily squeeze in and require the least amount of effort. Instead of "I will exercise for two hours a day," convenience says, "I will extend my workout for ten extra minutes a day" or "I will exercise one more day a week by walking or biking to the market instead of driving."

Habitual: All goals should break down into feasible habits. If, for example, the goal is to manage stress, break it down into specific habits like "first thing in the morning, I will take three large, calming breaths before I get up out of bed" and/or "before going to sleep, I will spend one minute identifying the best part of my day."

Infinitesimal: The smaller the habit, the easier it is to achieve. Losing weight sounds insurmountable to many people. But breaking that down into habits like: putting down the fork in between bites, swapping out a soda for a glass of water, stopping and assessing for true hunger before eating, and/or tracking daily intake by keeping a food journal are far more manageable.

Effortless: Similarly, the easier the habit, the more likely we will be able to incorporate it into a routine. If, for example, your goal is to eliminate using sugar in your morning cup of coffee, your morning routine need not change while your taste buds adjust to the less sweet cup of Joe. Or, if your aim is to eat more wholesome grains, you can swap in brown rice for white rice and whole-grain pasta for white pasta.

Victorious: Achievements are to be applauded. All of your victories, regardless of how large or small, should be celebrated. Putting down your fork when you're no longer hungry deserves a pat on the back—maybe even a happy dance. A great workout merits a few minutes reading a fun magazine—the effort acknowledged, and the behavior reinforced.

Exact: Specificity is a key element to achieving goals and habits. You can create infinite possible habits from wanting to "exercise more," for example. Instead, try exact specifies: "I will do thirty minutes of walking, three times a week starting after work at 4:30 p.m. on Mondays, Wednesdays, and Fridays and then perform thirty minutes of resistance training on Tuesdays and Thursdays also at 4:30 p.m., alternating upper body and lower body on either day." When the details are targeted, your goal can easily be scheduled into the calendar and on the road to settling in as a regular habit.

The Five Tools to Help ACHIEVE Goals and Habits

Once you've established your goals and habits, these five tools will help you implement and maintain them: lists, food journals, schedules, stocking up, and prepping.

1. LISTS

Lists can help to keep you organized and accountable. Many types of lists can be valuable when healthifying life, including:

- Goals and habits lists: Clarifying goals and habits and then writing them down, in a very visible place, as a regular reminder solidifies their existence. When they are displayed on paper (or pop up on your computer through a website or app), they become more tangible, accessible, present, and hard to ignore.
- Shopping lists: Going food shopping without a list is like driving somewhere new without directions. It promotes impulse buying, inefficient purchasing, and the need to return to the store more frequently than anticipated. Planning recipes and checking for ingredients you need simplifies food preparation. Keeping an ongoing list of staples as they are depleted ensures a well-stocked kitchen, alleviating some food prep tension and last minute scrambling.

- Recipe lists: Building a repertoire of healthful, Vegiterranean meals with fabulous recipes can really help you—and your family. The recipes in Chapter 9 are a great start—they are easy and friendly to a wide range of palates (adult and kid!). You can also find recipes online, in books, or in magazines. Maintaining a list or keeping the recipes in a single place gives you easy access for meal-planning.

2. FOOD JOURNALS

I recommend keeping a food journal to all of my clients. Tracking food intake, any symptoms, hunger/satiety levels, estimated portion sizes, weight, exercise performed, and/or emotions is the most effective way to stay accountable to choices and to determine what works versus what does not work. If, for example, you have problems with unexplained occasional indigestion, tracking those symptoms along with your food intake is the best way to find out what may be causing your issues. Or, if you want to lose weight, keeping tabs on not only your weight but also on the food you eat, hunger/satiety levels, and portion sizes can pinpoint which habits are helping and which may not be working. This can be on paper, in a dedicated notebook, online, in a document on the computer, using a specialized app—the key is making it easy to record. Many Websites and apps have revolutionized this habit of helping track food intake by including total calories in and out, calculating goal calories, acting as a pedometer, providing social support, and more.

3. SCHEDULES

Another blessing of modern technology is the ability to effectively maintain schedules. From a computer to a phone and back again, scheduling can get pretty high tech. My traditional self happens still to prefer writing it down on a monthly calendar so I can actually see it. But regardless of *how* you schedule, being adamant about doing so is one of the keys to success. To implement goals and behaviors, scheduling them in helps make them official. You can schedule success by inputting workouts, food shopping and prep time, appointments for relaxation time, and time for social support. While it might seem odd to schedule all of these things, it will help you to make sure you do them! You can schedule weeks or months in advance when possible, and prioritize goals and habits. If you fly a lot, you know what the flight attendants say before takeoff: Put your own oxygen mask on before assisting someone else. If you fail to take care of yourself first, you won't be effective at taking care of anyone or anything else.

4. STOCKING UP

A well-stocked kitchen is essential. With the constant accessibility of health-damaging foods at restaurants, markets, and even gas stations, your home needs to be a refuge for all things healthful. When you have delicious, nutritious staples in the pantry, fridge, and freezer, and simple equipment to whip them together into fully loaded meals, you will crave eating at home and will enjoy the luxury—trust me! The basic tools of the trade include appliances, utensils, gadgets, and food staples. You'll find more info on stocking your kitchen and pantry in the next chapter.

5. PREPPING

If you think you have to be an experienced chef to succeed at Vegiterraneanism, think again! Prepping and cooking food can be easy and doable for anyone and everyone. Investing a bit of time prepping items once or twice a week can make meeting habits and goals markedly easier. Spending time after returning home from grocery shopping or the farmers' market to wash and chop your produce makes cooking much easier. Having fresh, clean, chopped fruits and veggies ready to grab makes it much more convenient to make good choices. At the same time, also throwing together a large basic salad, a huge pot of soup, a bottle of homemade dressing, and some bean dip will serve well for at least four or five days. You can accomplish all of this in an hour or two, especially after you've set your routine.

Also in the prep category is deciding ahead of time which recipes to prepare for the week. Taking just a few minutes to map out the day or the week is a great investment in time, keeping life easy. The benefit of having a well-stocked kitchen, however, is being able to whip up a meal on a whim if a time-crunch didn't allow for planning.

STRATEGIZING ON THE GO

Now that you have some tools to work with, you can explore options for taking these ideas outside of your home. Dining out and traveling bring about a bit of challenge to sticking to healthy habits. Breaking routine can throw things awry, but with a bit of preparation and forethought, you can overcome and rise to the opportunity.

DINING OUT

Maintaining a health-promoting diet is much easier with full control over the kitchen. When venturing into someone else's kitchen, however, most bets are off. Yet, dining out and eating at gatherings of friends and relatives is pleasurable, relaxing, and an important part of living in society, and it is by no means mandatory to become a recluse in order to sustain a healthy diet. No opportunity is impossible to navigate with a bit of preparation, an optimistic attitude, and some careful consideration. Because the premise of the Vegiterranean Diet is to eat a wide variety of whole, plant foods, a mountain of options remains readily accessible no matter where you find yourself. Here is how to troubleshoot the dining experience:

Choose wisely: If having some control over the decision of where you are dining is possible, a frequented safe spot makes a great location. When widening the scope of restaurant-finding possibilities, a restaurant-finding Website or app, like HappyCow,[2] can suggest plant-friendly options locally, wherever that happens to be. These digital apps use GPS locating or provided addresses to suggest nearby options for various cuisines. Plus, these apps work around the globe so this is an ideal tool for travel, as well.

Check the menu ahead of time: Many events, business meetings, or other occasions, don't allow you to have a choice in the particular eating

Ethnic cuisine is far more likely to carry many more options for Vegiterraneans than an American-style abode. Most countries are traditionally plant-based and center their meals on grains, legumes, and vegetables. The delicious diversity of a new, never previously experienced cuisine like Ethiopian, Indian, or Vietnamese is worth the experiment.

VEGI-SIDE

establishment. Still, a little pre-meal investigating can prove helpful. If the restaurant is disclosed in advance, try to scope out the menu online; if the menu's not available, call ahead and ask questions. Many times, restaurant hosts or other staff will try and assist with dietary guidelines when provided. In certain areas, wait staff are used to these requests, especially with the amplified incidence of food allergies and intolerances increasingly common in the past couple of decades. When discussing whole plant options, you eliminate confusion by mentioning specifics (no meats, eggs, dairy, etc.). Telling the restaurant when the meal is scheduled and asking gently for a hearty meal with tons of vegetables, fruits, whole grains, beans, and lentils may result in a delicious experience. Mostly all restaurants carry staple items (perhaps to use as a garnish or side dish, in some less-than-ideal situations) like baked potatoes, rice, pasta, salad, and steamed veggies.

Expect the unexpected: Of course, situations will arise when neither time nor opportunity allow for advanced planning. No need to fear as a healthful meal can be pulled together anywhere. Granted, some places will provide more delicious and substantial options while others may look more like the worst-case scenario of boring, unsatisfying rabbit food. However, once you get used to dining out and planning ahead, you'll know that this is an abnormal instance, reasons other than the food brought you there, and you simply need to eat to fill yourself up enough to last until you can get away to a more satisfying meal. Surprisingly, it is pretty typical for restaurants to have items not listed on their menu, so it never hurts to dig deeper and ask your server. On a recent trip, I found myself with a seemingly insurmountable menu. At my request, the head chef came out to speak with me. After spending several minutes discussing my preferences and what he had available in the kitchen, he ended up serving me a memorably creative and delicious meal. The more you practice, the less of an obstacle dining out becomes.

PLOTTING A MEAL

Once you have sat down at a restaurant, you need to put on your plant goggles and scope out the menu prudently. If options are not immediately obvious, then you need to look more closely. Take a look at accompaniments and side dishes; these hint at what items are stocked in the kitchen and ready for use. For example, if potatoes, kale, or beans are side dishes or garnishes, that means they have those to serve, and you can kindly ask to have them made in a more main attraction sort of fashion.

In the most difficult situations (steakhouses and the like), creativity is key. You can think about the ingredients and what you would make with them; then, you can ask if it is possible. Almost like a puzzle: The restaurant serves steamed spinach, pasta, parsley, tomatoes, white beans, baked potatoes, and lemon wedges. How can you put it together? Therein lies the meal.

If the waitstaff make it difficult or are uninterested in meeting your needs, you need to get as simple as possible. A side of rice, a green salad, a balsamic vinegar, or a lemon wedge will have to do; still, this extreme experience is temporary and very rare. Typically, restaurants are eager to make patrons happy and help find a solution. You simply need to identify the ingredients you want and then order them. Next time, choose a different venue.

BEING A GUEST IN SOMEONE ELSE'S HOME

Of course, dining out is slightly different than heading over to a buddy's or relative's home for a meal. This can be an easier or a more challenging situation, depending on the buddy or the relative. Most importantly, you should remain prepared.

Best-case scenario: Your host knows you eat a whole food, plant-based Vegiterranean diet and she lets you know that the meal will be specifically tailored to your needs. You can ask what you can contribute to the meal so you know you have a solid dish to enjoy and share with others. A favorite dish not only guarantees something reliable to eat but may well inspire others, who will realize that this way of eating is delicious and keeps bodies feeling fab. Win others' hearts through their stomachs, as the old adage goes . . .

Or: Unfortunately, you'll probably find yourself in situations where your host knows you eat a whole food, plant-based Vegiterranean diet... but she lets you know ahead of time that the meal will certainly not address those needs. Your host may ask you to bring something yourself if you want an appropriate option. Cooking up a dish or two (or purchasing prepared foods to take, if preferred) is comforting, enabling reassurance that you will definitely have something you love to eat.

If you're not sure if your host is aware of your plant-based diet, call ahead and have an honest discussion. You can then best plan ahead so that you and your host have a good time. If that's not an option, here are two more suggestions:

- Eat beforehand and bring a dish along, just in case.
- In instances where there really is very little to eat, you just need to do your best with what is available until you can get to your next satisfying meal. While this isn't ideal, usually it's unintentional oversight on the host's part, so do your best to remain pleasant and gracious.

Ultimately, planning perseveres—fail to plan and plan to fail. You can take care of yourself by making sure you always have healthful, delicious food to eat as often as possible. This commitment to yourself is worth the small investment because of the benefits you reap. Compassion, of course, is always to be remembered . . . to yourself and to your hosts.

There's one surefire way of having delicious Vegiterranean options: Entertaining in your own home and inviting friends and family to enjoy a meal with you can be fantastic! This is one of the greatest ways to inspire and bond with others over the nutritious, decadent spread of Vegiterranean fare. Whenever I have guests, I make a buffet filled with variety, abundance, and my favorite, well-tested recipes. Nothing is more gratifying than having guests repeatedly ask: "*This* is healthy?!" or "*This* is vegan??" as it is proof positive that delicious makes nutritious achievable.

TRAVELING

If you're a Vegiterranean on the go, you'll want to really research and plan ahead in order to ensure an adequate supply of healthy food throughout your journeys. Carefully plotting for how long you'll need to be stocked up from door to door, as well as determining where you'll be able to find food while traveling, makes the process less stressful. Most of what you can bring along will depend on how you are traveling ... by car or by plane. Two of the biggest considerations are whether a cooler can be taken and, if flying, going through security.

The first step is figuring out how long you'll need supplies in order to get from home to your destination. Packing enough food to get through that leg of the trip keeps you from having to eat airport/airline foods or truck stop/fast food along the way. When traveling with others, bringing along enough food for yourself and your traveling companions is a good idea.

Flying eliminates the possibility for soups, smoothies, and pressed juices. Plenty of dried good and whole foods are options, but water will have to be purchased after going through airport security. Another more cost-effective and eco-friendly option is to take an empty stainless steel or BPA-free plastic water bottle to the airport, and then filling it up once you're cleared into the terminal.

Driving makes food accessibility far easier because you can pack however much you can squeeze into your car, and you can easily bring coolers to keep foods longer. Planning ahead and packing up plenty of food ensures you have lots of healthy options along the road.

Once you arrive at your destination, it all depends on how plant-friendly the location itself is. This is when those healthy food-finding apps and Websites, like HappyCow, come in super handy, as they can locate veg-friendly dining and markets just about anywhere. You can hit the market to stock up on some items for meals and snacks can supplement your packed foods. When staying with friends or family members, simply ask ahead if you can store some food in the fridge. When staying at a hotel, you can call ahead of time and request a refrigerator unit in the room. Most hotels will provide one. If not, you can use the ice bucket to keep perishables over ice, changing it regularly before it melts.

International travel can require even more planning. Be sure to research online ahead of time. When traveling to other countries, asking detailed questions may require a translation dictionary if a language barrier exists, so prepare before you pack up your passport! Most restaurants want to please their guests, and will go out of their way to accommodate patrons, even if you don't speak the same language.

Travel-Friendly Foods, Cooler-dependent Foods

- Salads in disposable containers with dressing in a separate container
- Fruits: whole, cut, salad, dried, dehydrated
- Baked potatoes, sweet potatoes, yams
- Hummus with chopped veggies and whole-grain crackers to dip
- Wraps or sandwiches made on whole-grain breads or tortillas with hummus or bean spread and veggies or nut or seed butter and whole-fruit jam or sliced fruits
- Edamame
- Veggie sushi
- Bean, rice, and veggie burritos with salsa and guacamole on the side and separate
- Whole-grain pasta with sauce
- Unopened precooked tempeh or tofu packages
- Leftovers packed in a disposable container
- Takeout from a healthy restaurant or market, packed in a disposable container

Easy Foods That Require No Refrigeration

- Dried oatmeal in separate baggies with seeds (chia, flax, hemp) and/or nuts (you can easily add hot water in your hotel room)
- Kale chips
- Whole-fruit and nut bars
- Baked bars, whole-food cookies, muffins, and whole-grain breads
- Whole-grain or raw crackers, breads, tortillas, bagels
- Dehydrated bean and veggie soups
- Nut butters
- Trail mix
- Jarred bean dips
- Nutritional yeast and other spices in individually wrapped baggies to bring to restaurants
- Dehydrated green juice powders (for times when you don't know when you'll find your next greens)

CHAPTER 8

Un Giorno Nella Vita ...

The Vegiterranean Kitchen

Like most things in life, food represents a spectrum from super simple to extravagant. Eating a Vegiterranean diet does not require much and Vegiterraneans can absolutely thrive without gourmet cuisine, special ingredients, or un-tasty essentials. Using the Vegiterranean Food Pyramid and Veg Ten as a guideline, personal style can then be added to the mix. The following equipment, fundamental foods, staples, storage, and swapping out ingredients are just some of the many possible recommendations on how to stay ready on the home front.

Appropriate Appliances

A kitchen equipped with the basics will keep you happily cooking: a functional stovetop and oven, along with a blender and a food processor, will help with easy meals. Here are some details on these helpful appliances.

High-powered blender: Blenders range from simple and small to powerful and large. High-powered blenders can liquefy anything in speedy seconds and are also equipped to heat up, to make simple soups and sauces. I splurged on one of these blenders a few years ago, and it is the best culinary investment I have made thus far, as I use it at least once or twice a day.

In this chapter you'll learn...
- Essential kitchen tools and gadgets
- How to stock your Vegiterranean pantry, fridge, and freezer
- The outs-and-ins of swapping conventional ingredients for Veg-friendly ones
- Easy oil-free food prep

Immersion blender: I used to make super smoothies with a simple immersion blender—a hand-held stick-like blender—that is much more cost-effective and easier to store. Immersion blenders make it easier to puree soups directly in the pot, without the splatter danger of transferring hot liquids to and from a standard blender.

Fruit and vegetable juicer: Extracting fresh juices from fruits and vegetables are excellent for fresh and nutritious beverages and also to use in recipes to add nutrient density a la a multivitamin in a glass. Kicking off your day with a green juice (or a green smoothie from the blender) on an empty stomach is an incredibly healthy habit. My favorite combinations include a base of cucumber with kale or other fresh greens, and a bit of ginger, lemon, carrot and/or some fresh melon or pineapple.

Food processor: These come in different sizes, and a bigger version may be best when you're cooking for more than one or two people. A food processor chops, purees, slices, dices, juliennes, and shreds, and, in my humble hummus-aficionado opinion, they enable the best texture for hummus, a Vegiterranean's best friend.

Rice cooker/steamer: With one of these, worrying about burning the bottom or monitoring the time becomes a thing of the past when cooking whole grains. It's so simple to set the rice cooker with the accurate ratio of water to grains, and let it slowly prepare a perfect product while creating the rest of the meal or going about your day. Bonus: It keeps the grains warm until turned off, leaving less pressure for time. Throwing some veggies in there at the end of cooking makes for a double bonus.

Slow cooker: This little appliance also enables "setting it and forgetting it" type cooking for the busy chef. You can throw ingredients together in the morning, turn the switch on, and dinner will be ready and waiting at mealtime.

Pressure cooker: This smart cooker can take dried beans and cook them within just a very short time! In literally minutes, soups, stews, beans, and more are done.

Dehydrator: Without a versatile oven that cooks at very low temperatures, it is tricky to make stellar kale chips or raw crackers without this fun accessory. However, a dehydrator can take up a bunch of counter space. If you use them, dehydrators are worth the investment of space and cost because you can make affordable dried fruits and vegetables. Also, soaking and dehydrating nuts, seeds, grains, and legumes helps to enhance the nutrient bioavailability, which improves their absorption.

Instant hot water dispenser: Should this fit in your kitchen and budget, you won't regret it. Having hot water ready-to-go is a worthy, fabulous frill!

Useful Utensils

You don't have to break the bank on outfitting your kitchen. Starting with the basics, suitable cookware and utensils can easily be selected and used for many years.

Cookware: Ceramic and stainless steel (that is not coated with another metal alloy) are the best types of cookware because they do not leech harmful metals into food, and food does not usually stick to them. Because most nonstick coatings contain toxins that are released when utensils scratch the surfaces, this type of cookware should be avoided. Some companies are producing eco-friendly, nontoxic products that may be worth exploring. You could easily get away with just one large saucepot (at least four quarts) and, perhaps, have a smaller-sized (two quart) saucepot for quicker cooking and easier cleanup. A large stockpot (approximately eight quarts) is excellent for making stocks, broths, soups, and stews. Then, it is ideal to have a large (about twelve inches in diameter) frying pan and a smaller one (approximately eight inches in diameter). If you typically cook for more people or in larger batches, you may want to build a larger collection so you can cook multiple dishes at once.

Bakeware: I highly recommend silicone bakeware for the same reasons noted above. Silicone is inert which means it won't interact with the food with which it comes into contact. Plus, silicone bakeware comes in various sizes, shapes, and colors. You can find loaf pans, square pans, baking pan liners (referred to as Silpat® liners), muffin "tins," and much more, and they are widely available in grocers' stores, kitchen stores, and online. Good basics to have on hand include a large roasting pan or casserole dish, a square 9 x 9-inch baking dish, a loaf pan, muffin tins, at least two baking sheets, and a couple of liners.

Storage containers: A good, varied set of glass or silicone storage containers is also essential for storing food and maintaining freshness. A collection of glass bowls, both large and small, is likewise necessary for mixing and serving. Glass mason jars are excellent for storage. Here's a good recycling tip: As ingredients that are sold in glass jars are depleted, the containers can be washed well and saved to use for storage. Tall, narrow-necked jars are great to store freshly made dressings and sauces while short, broader jars can be used to store foods bought in the bulk section at the market.

> Parchment paper also works as a liner on baking sheets to protect food from direct contact with metals.

Knives and a cutting board: A sturdy chef's knife to chop away at all those vibrant veggies, a serrated bread knife for careful cutting of tomatoes and bread, a paring knife, and an effective knife sharpener are the top four necessities in knives. Also, sharp scissors make quick work of chopping herbs; a second pair for opening packages will prevent cross-contamination. A healthy, stable cutting board choice is bamboo because the material is sustainable and, unlike plastic, free from chemicals.

Go-To Gadgets

Small must-haves include: glass or stainless steel measuring cups and spoons, a can opener, peeler, zester or microplane, grater, colander, large wooden spoons, spatulas, tongs, ladles, cheese cloth or mesh bag, garlic press, ice cream scoops for equal portioning, wooden citrus reamer or citrus press, whisks, rolling pin, and oven mitts. If you want to get a bit fancy, specialized kitchen apparatuses include:

- Apple corer: not just for apples, this handy tool assists with coring pears, oranges, pumpkins, and other produce
- Milk frother to make frothy beverages
- Spiral slicer or spiralizer to make thin ribbons of raw vegetables like cucumber, daikon radish, squash, sweet potato, and zucchini

- Mezzaluna, a half-moon-shaped knife, for easy rough chopping of vegetables like kale
- Melon baller to scoop fruit, baked potatoes, and other fruits and veggies into small spheres
- Mandoline, a hand-held instrument for slicing produce from very thin to thicker pieces
- Tofu press to make tofu denser and heartier. (Freezing and thawing tofu before using will also accomplish this.)
- Veggie chopper for expedited, more controlled chopping

Whatever your kitchen looks like, starting with the basics and easing into Vegiterranean cooking will allow you to familiarize yourself with different methods of cooking and the use of new gadgets; you may find that staying minimalistic is the better strategy for you.

Plentiful Pantry

Pantry provisions vary depending on size, season, and preference. While this list of suggestions is by no means exhaustive, it serves as a baseline of items used often in Vegiterranean eating and beneficial to keep in stock.

A well-stocked Vegiterranean pantry might have any of the following foods:

- Gluten-free whole grains: amaranth, black forbidden rice, brown rice, buckwheat, millet, (gluten-free) oats, purple or red rice, quinoa, wild rice, teff
- Gluten-containing grains (for those not sensitive, allergic, or with Celiac disease): bulgur, couscous, pearled barley, spelt, wheat berries
- Xanthan gum and arrowroot for thickening
- Whole-grain pasta: brown rice, corn, quinoa, whole wheat
- Whole-grain crackers: corn, rice, 100-percent whole-wheat
- Whole flours: almond, chickpea, cornmeal, gluten-free baking blend, oat, whole wheat or spelt

- Legumes: any and all dried beans, including black, fava, kidney, pinto, red, white; peas (black-eyed, chickpeas, green split, yellow split), and lentils (beluga black, green, red)
- Canned goods (ideally salt-free and in BPA-free cans): beans, corn, fruit and vegetable purees (applesauce, pear, pumpkin, sweet potato), lentils, water chestnuts
- Jarred goods: artichoke hearts, hot sauce, marinara sauce, olives, roasted red bell peppers, salsas, tomato paste, tomato sauce, vegan worcestershire
- Aseptically packed goods: beans, plant milks, purees (pumpkin), crushed tomatoes, vegetable broth
- Unopened nuts (raw, unsalted), seeds, nut butters, and seed butters (especially tahini)
- Nutritional yeast: Nutritional yeast is a primary cultured yeast grown on sugarcane and beet molasses and is fortified with plenty of B vitamins. While, unlike other yeasts, it does not have leavening power, it adds a tangy, nutty, and cheesy flavor and texture when sprinkled on its own onto popcorn, salads, whole grains, or roasted vegetables and when mixed into sauces, hummus, pizza, casseroles, and stews.
- Vinegars: apple cider, balsamic, rice, red wine
- Dried spices and spice blends: for the recipes found in Vegiterranean cuisine, stock up on ground allspice, dried basil, bay leaves, black pepper, cayenne pepper, chili powder, ground chipotle powder, ground cinnamon, ground cumin, dill, garlic powder, Italian seasoning blend, mint, nutmeg, onion, oregano, sweet paprika and smoked paprika, parsley flakes, pumpkin pie spice blend, red pepper flakes, rosemary, sage, thyme, turmeric
- Dried fruit: coconut, currants, dates, raisins, sun-dried tomatoes (yep, they're a fruit)

VEGI-SIDE

For other Veg friendly dishes outside of the Vegiterranean genre, spice blends such as Chinese five-spice blend, curry powder, garam masala, herbes de Provence, jerk seasoning, pickling spice, quatre-epices, and zahtar help support delicious, flavorful meals.

- Sweeteners: 100-percent-pure maple syrup, blackstrap molasses, pure date paste and/or syrup
- Cacao nibs and cocoa powder

Storage Tips

In a cool, dark pantry, many staples, like whole grains and legumes, will last quite a while. To maintain freshness and avoid spoilage, expiration dates should be noted and bulk-section purchases labeled. FIFO—first in, first out—is a helpful storage management technique accomplished by simply putting new items behind the older ones. Here is how to store common items:

Whole grains: These need to be stored more carefully than refined versions because of the healthy oil found naturally within the germ. Fats are more sensitive to heat, light, and moisture, and rancidity happens quicker. Intact grains should be stored in airtight containers and can keep for up to six months in a cool, dry place or up to a year in the freezer.

Whole grain flours: These are even more susceptible to spoilage since the oils have been ground up, exposing them to oxygen. Pantry storage will keep whole-grain flours fresh for one to three months, but freezer storage maintains freshness for two to six months.

Beans: Dried beans last at least a year in dry storage and longer in cold. If they are stored in oxygen-removed containers, they have a shelf life of up to ten years! Canned beans last about a year but have expiration dates to help keep tabs. Cooked beans last about four to five days in an airtight container in the refrigerator.

Nuts: Nuts are at high risk of rancidity due to their high fat content. Rancidity is a generalized term for food spoilage which makes it undesirable and, more importantly, unsafe for consumption mostly due to

Oils are much more prone to rapid rancidity since it is pure fat and the processing of a food into an oil increases its exposure to oxygen. Although a change in flavor or smell may not always be recognized with rancidity, the food will still wreak havoc on the body. This is another reason to minimize intake of oils.

VEGI-SIDE

oxidation. Nuts retain their quality for about a year in the refrigerator, two years in the freezer, and four months in the pantry.

Full Fridge

Truly, the refrigerator is the epicenter of a healthful lifestyle, as it is where fresh lives. The fridge also stores ingredients, leftovers, and essentials for at least a few days. Fresh cannot be forgotten so close monitoring will prevent smell-detectable spoilage and maintain a natural flow.

- Fresh vegetables
- Fresh herbs such as basil, cilantro, dill, garlic, ginger root, Italian (or flat leaf) parsley, mint, oregano, rosemary, sage, and thyme
- Some fruits (berries, melons) and whole-fruit jam
- Salads
- Raw nuts (almond, Brazil nuts, cashews, pine nuts, walnuts)
- Seeds (chia, flax, hemp, pumpkin, sesame, sunflower)
- Nut and seed butters (sunflower seed butter, tahini)
- Unsweetened (flavored or plain) plant milks: almond, hemp, oat, rice, soy
- Organic or specified non-GMO soy products: miso paste, tamari or Bragg liquid aminos, tempeh, tofu (silken, soft, firm, extra firm)
- Extracts: vanilla especially, but you may also enjoy using almond, coconut, peppermint, rose water, and other extracts (I prefer alcohol-free for enhanced flavor)
- Condiments: mustards (Dijon, spicy brown, yellow), ketchup, prepared horseradish, pure kosher dill pickles and pickle relish (all without sugar or preservatives), sauerkraut, vinegars (apple cider, balsamic, rice, red wine)

VEGI-SIDE

A good rule of thumb for fresh to dried herb/spice conversion in a recipe is that one tablespoon of fresh herbs is equivalent to one teaspoon dried.

Functional Freezer

Freezing foods and leftovers can be very efficient, helping to save time and costs by keeping food longer. Out-of-season foods (frozen when they *were* in season) become enjoyable year-round. Ready-to-go meals may be prepared in advance for those times when shopping and cooking isn't possible. Batch cooking and buying seasonal products at their peak freshness and lowest cost highlight the freezer's fabulousness. For example, I love Meyer lemons, but they are only available between December and April. When they are in season, I buy a ton of them, zest and juice them, and pop them in the freezer for a mid-year treat. Here are some freezer staples to keep on hand:

- Frozen bananas, berries, and other fruits (organic, when possible)
- Frozen vegetables: broccoli, corn, greens, mushrooms, peas, mixed blends
- Frozen herbs, garlic, ginger
- Precooked brown rice
- Whole fruit popsicles or sorbet

The Outs-and-Ins of Swapping

Eating a whole food, plant-based Vegiterranean diet means swapping out some usual basic ingredients. Some examples:

- Plant-based dairy alternatives for dairy products
- Natural plant thickeners and emulsifiers for gelatin
- Vegetable broth for animal-based broth
- Mushrooms, lentils, seitan, and soy products for meat
- Whole food sweeteners instead of sugars or artificial sweeteners

Fortunately, these substitutions have become so commonplace that it is easy to find all of these ingredients in most grocery stores, health food shops, and multiple venues online that ship them straight to the door, for added convenience. Further, to save money and to have full control of all ingredients going into our bodies, we can effortlessly make most of these foods at home!

Plant Milks

It may be hard to miss the wall-o'-plant milks currently taking up major amounts of real estate in both the cold and dry shelf spaces at the grocery store. Of the myriad choices, "milks" are made of almond, hemp, soy, oat, rice, flax, and coconut. If that weren't exciting enough, flavored versions such as vanilla, chocolate, pumpkin, chai, eggnog, chocolate peppermint, and more are available. Granted, many of these fancier beverages are loaded with sugars so they are not ideal options for most of us. Each of these milks have distinctive qualities that provide unique culinary and flavor opportunities. Soy and coconut are velvety and smooth, perfect for coffee, tea, smoothies, and blended ice creams. Hemp and oat milks are a bit grainier and go well in whole-grain cereals, smoothies, or soups. Almond is light, creamy, and neutral-flavored and works in any recipe that can handle a subtle nutty tone. Flax is slightly oily and has a distinct flavor so testing this plant milk separately before committing to using it in a recipe is a good idea. Plenty of variety can be found in the plant milk category, and selecting unsweetened varieties to avoid added sugars is really the only caveat.

VEGI-SIDE

Homemade plant milks do not contain the fortified nutrients like store-bought versions so consuming calcium and vitamin D from other sources is required.

We can also make our own plant milks at home by blending water with nuts, seeds, rice, or soybeans and then straining out the pulp with specialized nut milk bags (or a plain old paint straining bag works just as well, but for a fraction of the cost). See Chapter 9 for a detailed recipe.

Dairy-Free Deliciousness

Varieties of commercially made plant-based cheeses, cream cheeses, ice creams, and other dairy alternatives are rapidly increasing in the marketplace, which is an excellent sign of the times. Nonetheless, as manufacturers try to provide healthier substitutes for the dairy products with which most of us grew up, many of these alternatives use oils and other additives to achieve similar properties. When selecting from the many products, those with the fewest additives are better choices, or we could consider making our own to guarantee wholesomeness. In addition to a growing list of new products in stores, some extraordinary cookbooks and online recipes for DIY (do-it-yourself) options made from whole plant elements allow us to maintain control—and these foods taste divine.

Ingredients that impart a cheesy flavor include nutritional yeast, miso paste (a salty, pungent fermented soybean paste originally from Japan), and certain combinations of foods such as onion powder, garlic powder, arrowroot, nutritional yeast, roasted red peppers, cooked potatoes, beans, nuts, seeds, or whole-grain flours. Yes, we can have our cheese and eat it, too, but *sans* hormones and saturated fats that come in the original! We can experiment with some of these delicious approaches, adding our favorites to our Vegiterranean recipe boxes. You'll find easy, DIY dairy alternative recipes on pages 185–186.

Egg Substitutes

Not only are eggs merely eaten on their own, they are used for various purposes in cooking and baking. Eggs bind, leaven, and thicken, as well as increase volume, richness, and tenderness due to their especially high protein and fat content. Fortunately, these properties are easily replaced by using healthier, cholesterol-free, plant alternatives, specific to the called-for needs of the type of dish being prepared.

Assorted commercial egg replacers are available in stores and online. Typically, they come as neutrally flavored powders, and, therefore, are suitable for both savory and sweet dishes. Brands like Ener-G and Bob's Red Mill call for 2 tablespoons of warm water per 1 1/2 teaspoons of egg replacer to equal one egg in a recipe, but package directions should always be followed specifically.

For binding in baked goods, one egg can be replaced with 2 tablespoons cornstarch, arrowroot, or the miraculous flax egg. To prepare the flax egg replacement, 1 tablespoon ground flaxseeds should be blended or whisked with 3 tablespoons water, then set aside to watch the magic happen. After a few short minutes, a thick, white, omega-3-fat-rich, very inexpensive, versatile flax egg is ready to add to a recipe. Chia seeds act similarly, except because they absorb exponentially more water, the ratio is 1 teaspoon of chia seeds per 3 tablespoons of water; the chia seeds do not need to be ground.

Other egg replacers that work wonders in baked recipes are fruit and vegetable purees, adding moisture and boosting nutrition. For the equivalent of one egg, one-half banana, mashed, or one-quarter cup pureed fruits (e.g., applesauce, prunes) or vegetables (e.g., pumpkin, sweet potato) can be substituted.

Finally, the incredibly multitalented tofu can be swapped in for eggs in scrambles, quiches, frittatas, egg salads, and more. A bit of turmeric adds natural (phytochemical-rich) yellow coloring in these recipes. For egg-like flavoring, onion powder, garlic powder, paprika, and nutritional yeast can mimic the taste. Silken tofu will add creamy thickness without altering the flavor of a dish, and it is also works to make puddings, mayonnaise, sauces, and dressings.

Mock Meats

Like dairy alternatives, meat analogues are also rapidly moving into grocery stores and restaurants everywhere. Faux forms of everything from turkey and shrimp to ground round and chicken nuggets are readily available. Although these are not exactly *whole* plant foods, they serve a couple important purposes. First, they help people transition from the meat-and-potatoes standard American diet—which is how most of us were raised—to a healthier, more sustainable and compassionate lifestyle, offering similar flavors and textures without health-damaging hormones, saturated fats, antibiotics, heme iron, and the like found in the animal versions. Secondly, they bridge the gap for people wanting to include these types of foods in their diets or under certain circumstances. For example, kids can have plant versions of similar foods such as "chicken" nuggets or a "turkey" sandwich when they are with friends or at parties so they don't feel left out. Or, we can enjoy a festive faux "turkey" at Thanksgiving. You may well find, though, that you prefer simply avoiding anything meat-like or as your taste buds adjust, you may want to treat them as an occasional indulgence or do away with them altogether.

For more wholesome, densely textured meat alternatives, seasoned, cooked mushrooms, tempeh, extra-firm tofu, and/or lentils can replace whole or coarsely ground meats. Grilled portabello mushroom caps can serve as substitutes for burgers or in other sandwiches. Seitan—affectionately known as "wheat meat," as it is made from gluten, the protein in wheat—works well when cooked and added to stews, sautés, or flavored on its own.

Other Plant Swaps

Other recipe ingredients that can easily be switched out include the following:

- Broth: equal parts vegetable broth exchanged for animal-based broth
- Gelatin: 1 tablespoon can be replaced with 1 tablespoon of agar agar flakes (a gelatinous sea vegetable that thickens in water) or 1/2 teaspoon agar powder
- Gelling agents: arrowroot, chia seeds, cornstarch, guar gum, tapioca starch, and xanthan gum can all be used to thicken soups, sauces, puddings, custards, jellies, and dressings (Follow instructions in recipes for appropriate ratios.)
- Frozen dessert: make your own plant-based ice cream with frozen fruits blended alone or with cacao powder, nut butter, unsweetened shredded coconut and/or seeds (sometimes a splash of plant milk helps make the blender whir)
- Honey or agave: maple syrup or date paste (see page 184 for recipe)

Oil-Free Cooking

Swapping out oils from your cooking for the multiple health benefits explored throughout the book requires a simple switch in cookery technique. Once you start preparing foods without oil, it will become second nature and you will recognize how little you miss it. Here is what you need to know to get started:

- The correct cookware for oil-free cooking is, ideally, the type that food does not usually stick to. Ceramic and stainless steel have that capability and have the added bonus of being the safest types, too.
- For the most successful, slippery, non-toxic, nonstick baking, the best choice is silicone bakeware. As mentioned earlier, silicone is an inert compound and will, therefore, not leech into food or emit fumes or pose health risks. Products come in every shape and size imaginable (and then some), and silicone liners to use with other types of baking sheets are available, as well. Silicone tolerates both high and low temperatures so it can be transferred from fridge to oven or in reverse.
- Cooking oil-free is a humble art that is easily adopted. Typically, oil is used in sautéing or as an ingredient. For stovetop cooking, oil can be swapped out for water, vegetable stock, vinegar, pure juice, tea, coconut water, wine, beer, or plant milks. Typically, more liquid is needed than recommended in a recipe when replacing oil. If a recipe calls for a tablespoon of oil, one-quarter cup of replacement liquid is a common equivalent. The trick is to monitor food closely as it cooks to ensure it stays moist and is continuously moving.
- In sauces or dressings, oil can be used for flavor, creaminess, or moisture. Flavor can, instead, be incorporated with fresh herbs, spices, vinegars, and extracts. Flaxseeds, hempseeds, chia seeds, plant milks, silken tofu, or cannellini beans make good substitutes to achieve creaminess. To boost moisture, a recipe may be infused with water, vegetable stock, tomato sauce, plant milks, tea, wine, beer, or pure juice.
- Baking oil-free is more technical since baking is quite a precarious science. Generally speaking, substituting half of the amount of oil or margarine called for in a recipe with applesauce, mashed banana, pureed fruit or vegetable, silken or soft tofu, or mashed avocado works, depending on the flavor profile of the food prepared.

CHAPTER 9

Buon Appetito!

The Recipes

Here come the recipes! From light morning fare through hearty, satiating dinners, sweet indulgent desserts to savvy snacks, enjoying the culinary journey through the Med is to taste how divine Vegiterraneanism is ...

Many of these dishes were created with the help of my Mediterranean mother-in-law, Miri, as we happily healthified classic recipes. But I also am honored to include a handful of original recipes from the extraordinary culinary geniuses, Chad Sarno and Robin Robertson, along with some of my go-to quintessential staples. These meals may be enjoyed family-style or on their own, and feel free to be flexible with them. Personal preferences can—and should—absolutely be accommodated. Designed to be simple, delicious essentials and to create healthful options to eat anytime, these recipes can be tailored to suit any dietary needs. To sustained health and *buon appetito*!

Homemade Basics/Staples

Prepping basic staples at home is a great way to save cash, control flavor and ingredients, and avoid undesirable additives. Below are some basic recipes, made simple, for you to whip up in a flash using ingredients you likely have stocked up. Also included are some easy techniques for soaking and sprouting, to help boost nutrient absorption.

Parma Shake   *Makes 1 cup*

Blend up this shaker in just one minute, and use as Parmesan. Sprinkle it over pasta, salad, popcorn, or whole grains. Sea vegetable powder, granulated kelp, and dulse, or sea lettuce flakes, can be found in the spice aisle of your local grocery store, health food shops, or online.

    ½ cup raw nuts (almonds, cashews, Brazil nuts, or others) or hempseeds
    ½ cup nutritional yeast
    2 tablespoons raw sesame seeds
    1 teaspoon sea vegetable powder, nori, dulse, or wakame or ¼ teaspoon
        iodized salt

1. In a blender, process the nuts, nutritional yeast, sesame seeds, and sea vegetable powder briefly until well combined, 10 to 20 seconds.
2. Store in an airtight container in the refrigerator for up to 7 days.

Savory Sprinkles   *Makes 1½ cups*

Similar to the Parma Shake recipe, this cheesy substitute lends a savory and tangy taste because of the Mediterranean-flavored sun-dried tomatoes.

    ½ cup sun-dried tomatoes
    ½ cup hempseeds
    ½ cup nutritional yeast
    2 tablespoons sesame seeds (optional)

1. In a very dry blender, blend the sun-dried tomatoes until finely ground, 5 to 10 seconds.

2. Add the hempseeds, nutritional yeast, and sesame seeds to the blender, and blend only until well combined, 10 to 20 seconds.

3. Enjoy immediately or store in an airtight container in the refrigerator for up to a week.

Note: Do not let the blender heat up, or the ingredients will stick together and be difficult to remove from the container.

Betta' than Feta
Makes 1½ cups

Time to get your hands dirty and feel like a kid again! This recipe is so easy and fun, you can make it on a whim with staple ingredients in your kitchen. Turn a salad Greek, add it to a grain dish, or eat it on its own; this version is betta' than feta for your health.

3 tablespoons nutritional yeast
2 tablespoons freshly squeezed lemon juice with zest
1 tablespoon red wine vinegar
1 teaspoon dried basil
1 teaspoon dried rosemary
1 teaspoon dried oregano
1 (14-ounce) package extra-firm tofu

1. In a medium bowl, combine the nutritional yeast, lemon juice and zest, red wine vinegar, basil, rosemary, and oregano. Stir to combine. Crumble the tofu into the bowl, and stir or massage to combine.

2. Cover the bowl with plastic wrap and refrigerate to allow flavors to absorb, at least 1 hour. Serve immediately or store in an airtight container in the refrigerator for up to 3 or 4 days.

Bettermilk
Makes 1 cup

Does a favorite recipe call for buttermilk? Make it better with Bettermilk, sour and creamy, but healthy, too! Choose the type of plant milk according to what you will be using it for. Soymilk tends to be creamier and neutrally flavored, while almond and coconut milks have slight, but noticeable flavors, and rice milk tends to be thinner and grainier.

1 cup plant-based milk
2 teaspoons lemon or lime juice or white or cider vinegar

1. In a measuring cup or a bowl, combine the milk with the lemon juice and mix well. Let stand until curdled, 3 to 5 minutes. Use immediately.
Note: The recipe may be decreased or increased as needed.

Sour Tofu Cream   *Makes about 2 cups*

Whip up this rich, creamy, soy-based sour cream in a jiff to enjoy as a condiment or to use in recipes calling for sour cream.

1 (14-ounce) package silken or soft tofu
¼ cup plain, unsweetened plant-based milk
4 tablespoons freshly squeezed lemon juice
2 tablespoons nutritional yeast
1 tablespoon chopped fresh parsley or 1 teaspoon dried parsley flakes
1½ teaspoons sea vegetable powder, kelp, or dulse or ¼ teaspoon salt

1. In a food processor, process the tofu, milk, lemon juice, nutritional yeast, parsley, and sea vegetable powder until smooth, 30 to 60 seconds.
2. Serve immediately or store in an airtight container in the refrigerator for up to 4 to 5 days.

Date Paste   *Makes 1 cup*

Dried dates stay fresh in the pantry for quite a while, so having them on hand is a convenient way to replace added sugars in desserts, sauces, dressings, puddings, and more.

1 cup dried dates

1. In a small bowl, cover the dates with 1 cup water, or more as needed. Cover the bowl.
2. Allow the dates to soak in the refrigerator until they soften, at least 1 hour. Drain the dates and use as needed.

Basic Nut or Seed Milk   *Makes 3 to 4 cups*

Nut and seed milks are delicious beverages that are easy and cost-effec-tive to make yourself at home. Enjoy it in a glass, over cold cereal, or use it to sauté vegetables with, or to make a soup or stew creamy. Replace commercial versions in the recipes in this chapter, if you wish.

Note: I use a nut milk bag to strain my milks. You can find these at health food stores or online; you can also use the alternatives mentioned below to strain your milks.

> 1 cup raw nuts (almonds, cashews, hazelnuts, peanuts, pecans, pistachios, or walnuts) or seeds (hemp or sunflower)
> 3 cups water
> 1 to 2 tablespoons pure maple syrup or 2 to 3 pitted dates (optional)
> 1 teaspoon vanilla extract (optional)

1. Soak nuts or seeds in water, covered by at least a couple of inches, for at least 12 hours in a large bowl. Before preparing the nut milk, drain and rinse them well.

2. In a blender, process the nuts or seeds with the water, maple syrup or dates, and vanilla extract (if using) until smooth, approximately 1 minute.

3. Fit a nut milk bag, several layers of cheesecloth, a fine mesh sieve, or a paint-straining bag into a large bowl. Pour the milk through the strainer into the bowl, allowing the fiber to remain in the strainer. Squeeze the strainer or use a spatula or spoon to press the pulp and retrieve all of the liquid from the solids. The remaining pulp can be discarded, or, better yet, dehydrate the leftovers and use it in smoothies, as a healthy, crunchy top-ping over salads or desserts, or blended into a flour to use in recipes.

4. Enjoy immediately or store in an airtight container in the refrigera-tor for up to 4 to 5 days.

DIY Nut or Seed Butter   *Makes approximately 1½ cups*

Most commercial nut and seed butters are loaded with unhealthy addi-tives. What's nutty (hee-hee) is that making your own at home is perhaps one of the easiest swaps of all. Simply put, you can use most any nuts, seeds, or combinations you prefer into the food processor and process away. But bring your patience, as it requires several, super hypnotic minutes to smooth out. You can leave it as is or add a pinch of salt, and/or a dash of pure maple syrup at the end and then give it another quick whirl. If you are feeling extra creative or using the butter for a specific dish, you can add sweet ingredients such as vanilla extract, maple syrup, cinnamon, cacao powder, or make it savory with spices like chili powder, cumin, or garam masala. For a chunky version, take out about half a cup of the nuts before processing and add them back in at the end.

3 cups nuts (almonds, cashews, hazelnuts, peanuts, pecans, pistachios, or walnuts) or seeds (hemp or sunflower)
1 to 2 tablespoons pure maple syrup (optional)
Pinch of salt (optional)

1. In a food processor, process nuts or seeds. Initially, it forms a powder. At about 1 minute, the nuts or seeds start clumping together. After approximately 5 minutes, it starts to get creamier. But it takes at least 10 to 15 minutes (or more) to become smooth like butter. Make sure you keep going until it is smooth and velvety.

2. Add in maple syrup and salt if using. Store in an airtight container in the refrigerator for up to 1 week.

Prepping and Cooking Lentils

Lentils are available in dozens of varieties, ranging in size, color, shape, texture, and flavor. Three of the most popular varieties used in the U.S. are green, brown, and red, but a world of awesome options are available, like beluga black and yellow dal. Preparation of lentils includes picking out any small stones or debris, followed by a nice rinse in a strainer. Once rinsed, boiling lentils on a stovetop is simple. On average, 1 cup of lentils requires 3 cups of liquid (usually water or vegetable broth, depending on how they will be eaten). Bring the liquid to a boil in a medium saucepan over medium-high heat, and add lentils once it is boiling. Depending on their size, lentils require between 10 to 60 minutes of cooking. Green and brown lentils require longer, about 25 to 30 minutes, while red lentils can fully cook in closer to 15 to 20 minutes. If a mushier texture is desired (i.e., for mashing), they should cook a bit longer. Once cooked, lentils can be seasoned as desired, served, and/or used to complete the recipe.

Prepping and Cooking Beans

Beans differ from lentils in that they require presoaking and they need to cook longer than lentils. Soaking beans helps reduce cooking time, results in better end products, and also—perhaps most importantly—reduces the amount of gas-promoting oligosaccharides many people complain about from eating beans. Adding a strip of kombu seaweed to the pot during cooking helps reduce this effect as well. You can choose from three different ways to soak beans: quick soak, traditional soak, or hot soak. Traditional and hot soaking require preparation ahead of time.

Quick soak: For those days when you haven't planned ahead, you can use the quick soak method. In a large pot, place the beans along with water in a ratio of 5 cups water per cup of beans. Bring the water to a boil over medium-high heat and allow to cook for an additional 2 to 3 minutes. Turn off the heat, drain the beans, discard the cooking water, and rinse with fresh water before beginning the actual cooking process.

Traditional soak: Traditional soaking entails placing beans in a large bowl and covering with cold water. Cover and let sit in the refrigerator for at least 8 hours or overnight. Drain the beans, discard the soaking water, rinse with fresh water, and then cook as desired.

Hot soak: Finally, the hot soak method is perhaps the best method for reducing cooking time and producing tender beans.[1] First, place beans into a large pot with the ratio of 5 cups of water per cup of beans. Heat water to boiling and boil for an additional 2 to 3 minutes. Remove the beans from the heat, cover with a lid, and allow to stand for 2 to 24 hours. Drain the beans, discard the cooking water, rinse with fresh water, and begin the actual cooking process.

Cooking beans: Cooking beans is similar to cooking lentils. After presoaking and rinsing, place the beans in a large pot and add approximately 3 times the amount of water, or 3 cups water per 1 cup of beans.

Bring to a boil, keep lid tilted, and lower heat. Cook time depends on the size of the bean, the altitude, the age of the beans, the hardness of the water, and other factors so test with a fork often, add water as necessary, and cook until tender. Most beans take between forty and ninety minutes. Try adding aromatics like garlic cloves, a whole peeled onion, peppercorns, and/or bay leaves, but remove them when cooking is complete. Cooked beans can be stored in an airtight container in the refrigerator for up to three days and for several weeks or months in the freezer.

VEGI·SIDE

A quick-cook method includes using a pressure cooker, where lentils can be completely ready in 5 to 10 minutes and beans in 5 to 25, depending on the type!

Sprouting Legumes

Sprouts are superfoods. During the process of sprouting, significant changes occur in the plant that benefits the consumer. Anti-nutrients—compounds in plant foods that may inhibit absorption of micronutrients—are deactivated, enabling more nutrition to be absorbed from the food when eaten. Here's an easy method for sprouting legumes:

1. Wash and rinse legumes.

2. Place them into a large, clean glass jar and fill with water. For every ½ cup legumes, cover with approximately 3 inches of water. Cover with a piece of cheesecloth or muslin and secure with a rubber band, or use a mesh screen over the jar, and leave to soak for at least six hours or overnight.

3. Drain and discard soaking water and rinse sprouts two or three times. Once drained, return them to the jar, reseal, and turn the jar on its side; leave in a warm place (but away from direct sunlight).

4. Each day, rinse legumes well and return to jar to continue growing. Once sprouts start to show small green leaves and stems, after two to three days, rinse, and transfer into an airtight container. Enjoy immediately or keep stored in the fridge for up to three days.

Bevande (Beverages)

These satisfying blended beverages may be enjoyed first thing in the morning or as a meal during the day. They taste best when consumed immediately.

Brain-Boosting Blue Smoothie *Makes 2 cups*

This sweet and refreshing blue-licious beverage will bring on your inner brainiac with all those omega-3 fats and potent antioxidants.

1 cup unsweetened almond or other plant milk
1 cup packed chopped kale or other leafy green
½ cup frozen or fresh blueberries
½ medium-size banana, frozen (about ½ to 1 cup)
¼ cup hempseeds

1. Place the almond milk, kale, blueberries, banana, and hempseeds in a blender, and puree until smooth, 15 to 30 seconds.
2. Serve immediately.

Moroccan Mint Chia Tea *Makes 3 cups*

Morocco—one of the many countries bordering the Mediterranean—is famous for its traditional tea, steeped with plenty of fresh mint, known as *nana*, and sweetened. This blended version enables you to drink the healthy mint leaves and adds texture and satiety with chia seeds, making it a meal in and of itself.

2 cups brewed black or other tea, cooled well in the refrigerator
1 cup unsweetened almond or other plant milk
½ cup fresh mint leaves, stems removed
2 tablespoons pure maple syrup
2 tablespoons chia seeds

1. In a blender, puree the tea, almond milk, mint, and maple syrup until smooth, 10 to 20 seconds.

2. Stop the blender and add the chia seeds. Blend on a low speed just to mix in the seeds, 5 to 10 seconds.

3. Pour the tea into a glass and let sit until the chia seeds absorb the liquid and expand exponentially, 5 to 10 minutes.

Note: You may need to stir the tea before enjoying, as some of the seeds settle to the bottom.

Pumpkin Pie Green Smoothie   *Makes 2¼ cups*

Who needs the holidays for a sweet, spicy indulgence when it is jam-packed with immune-boosting carotenoids? This classic spicy-sweet combo tastes just like pumpkin pie in a glass—with the added bonus of greens!

1 cup unsweetened almond, soy, or other plant milk
1 cup packed fresh spinach leaves
1 cup frozen mango chunks
½ cup canned pumpkin puree (not pumpkin *pie* puree)
2 tablespoons pure maple syrup
1 teaspoon pumpkin pie spice

1. Combine the almond milk, spinach, mango, pumpkin puree, maple syrup, and pumpkin pie spice in a blender, and puree until smooth, 10 to 20 seconds.

2. Serve immediately.

Vegiterranean Athlete's Drink   *Makes 1 liter (or just over 1 quart)*

Here is a delicious, natural sports drink recipe that will help sustain you during endurance activities:

4 cups water, coconut water, and/or tea
¼ cup pitted dates or 100-percent-pure maple syrup
Freshly squeezed juice of 1 lemon, lime, or orange
¼ teaspoon salt

In a blender or food processor, combine the water, dates, lemon, lime, or orange juice, and salt. Blend on high until the dates are liquefied or until well combined, 10 seconds. Pour into a sports bottle(s) or store in the refrigerator in an airtight container for 4 to 5 days.

Salse e Condimenti per Insalata (Sauces, Spreads, and Dressings)

These recipes are versatile and universal in Vegiterranean foods. Use them as condiments on the side, as dips for vegetables, crackers, or breads, or as dressings over fresh vegetables or whole grains.

Tahina
Makes about 1¼ cups

Tahina is a staple in Middle Eastern cuisine, made with tahini (ground sesame paste) and served as a spread for pita and sandwiches, as a dipping sauce for foods like falafel, or as a sauce over whole grains and lentils.

1 cup tahini
½ cup fresh Italian flat-leaf parsley, leaves and stems
3 garlic cloves, minced
2 tablespoons freshly squeezed lemon juice with zest
½ teaspoon paprika or smoked paprika
¼ to ½ teaspoon salt

1. Using a standing blender or an immersion blender and a deep cup or jar, puree the tahini, 1 cup water, parsley, garlic, lemon juice and zest, paprika, and salt until very smooth, 10 to 20 seconds.

2. Serve immediately with additional paprika and chopped fresh parsley as a garnish, if desired, or store in an airtight container in the refrigerator for up to 4 or 5 days.

Note: To thin dressing, add additional water 1 teaspoon at a time until you reach desired consistency. To serve as a dip, make thicker by reducing the water.

Baba Ganoush

Makes 1½ cups

A very popular side dish in the Mediterranean, as well as in the Middle East, this broiled or roasted eggplant is cooked so the pulp becomes soft and smoky. Then, the eggplant—also called aubergine, a nightshade berry— is mashed, seasoned, and served as a dip with pita. Baba Ganoush is also fab on sandwiches, wraps, and veggie burgers, in salads, and with grains.

1 large eggplant
1 tablespoon freshly squeezed lemon juice with zest
¼ cup tahini
2 or 3 garlic cloves, minced
½ teaspoon crushed red pepper flakes
Pinch of salt (optional)

1. Preheat the oven to 400°F.
2. With a fork, poke several holes throughout the eggplant and place on a baking sheet lined with a silicone liner or parchment paper. Roast in the oven until skin appears darkened and wrinkled, about 30 minutes. Turn the eggplant over. Bake until the skin appears dark and crispy, 15 to 30 more minutes.
3. Split the eggplant, drain excess liquid, and scrape out the flesh into a bowl. Add remaining ingredients and mash together with a fork, until well-combined and creamy.
4. Serve immediately or store in an airtight container in the refrigerator for 3 to 4 days.

Hummus of the Earth

Makes 1¾ cups

Hummus should be a food group with its infinite combinations of ways to enjoy. With the addition of cannellini beans and spices, this essential version is earthy, warm, and classic. Use it in sandwiches, as a dip, or in salad.

2 cups cooked chickpeas, drained and rinsed if using canned
1 cup cooked cannellini beans, drained and rinsed if using canned
¼ cup nutritional yeast

1½ to 2 tablespoons freshly squeezed lemon juice with zest
1½ tablespoons tahini
1 tablespoon tamari
¾ teaspoon ground cumin
¾ teaspoon smoked paprika
¾ teaspoon ground chipotle powder
⅛ teaspoon crushed red pepper flakes

1. In a food processor, combine the chickpeas, cannellini beans, nutritional yeast, ¼ cup water, lemon juice and zest, tahini, tamari, cumin, paprika, chipotle powder, and red pepper flakes, and puree until smooth, 30 to 60 seconds, scraping down the sides of the bowl as needed.

2. Serve immediately or store in an airtight container in the refrigerator for 3 to 4 days.

Almond Sun-Dried Tomato Hummus   *Makes 2½ cups*

A tomato-infused hummus option to spice up those chickpeas, this dip is perfect for whole-grain breads and crackers. You can also use the Mediterranean-inspired array of flavors as a spread on sandwiches and wraps. Almond butter adds a richness and additional protein.

½ cup dry sun-dried tomatoes
2 (15-ounce) cans chickpeas, drained and rinsed
2 tablespoons almond butter
2 tablespoons freshly squeezed lemon juice with zest
1 teaspoon ground cumin
¼ teaspoon crushed red pepper flakes

1. In a very dry food processor fitted with an S blade, puree sun-dried tomatoes until well chopped, 10 to 20 seconds. Add chickpeas, 1/2 cup water, almond butter, lemon juice and zest, cumin, and red pepper flakes, and process until well-combined and smooth, 5 to 10 seconds.

2. Serve immediately with crudites or whole-grain crackers or as a sandwich spread. Or store in an airtight container in the refrigerator for up to 4 to 5 days.

Note: To thin, add more water, as desired.

White Bean and Rosemary Dip   *Makes 1½ cups*

A light and rustic dip that easily accompanies any meal, serve this creamy concoction with whole-grain bread, crudites, or whole-wheat pitas or as a sandwich spread.

¾ to 1 cup vegetable stock
2 garlic cloves, minced (optional)
1 tablespoon minced fresh rosemary
2 (15-ounce) cans cannellini (or other white) beans, drained and rinsed
2 teaspoons freshly squeezed lemon juice with zest
Pinch of salt and pepper, or more to taste

1. In a medium saucepan, bring the vegetable stock, garlic, and rosemary to a boil over medium-high heat until soft, about 5 minutes. Once hot, add the beans and reduce heat. Simmer over low heat until beans soften, 4 to 6 minutes. Add the lemon juice and zest, salt, and pepper and stir to combine.

2. With an immersion blender or transferred into a standing blender, puree until smooth, 5 to 10 seconds.

3. Serve immediately or store in an airtight container in the refrigerator for up to 4 or 5 days.

Smoky Avocado Dip   *Makes 2 to 4 servings*

Avocados are prepared simply, yet elegantly, with a subtle smoked, lemony flavor. Serve as a dip with toasted whole-grain pita or baked tortillas, or enjoy as a garnish with bean and rice or grain dishes.

2 medium-size ripe avocados, peeled, pitted and cut into chunks (1½ cups)
2 tablespoons freshly squeezed lemon juice with zest
¾ teaspoon smoked paprika (use sweet paprika if you prefer a more neutral flavor)
¼ teaspoon salt (optional)

1. In a small bowl, combine the avocados, lemon juice and zest, paprika, and salt, and stir until well mixed.

2. Serve immediately as it will turn brown rapidly.

Cashew Caesar Dressing
Makes 2 cups

RECIPE BY CHAD SARNO

This creamy and rich salad dressing is the perfect complement to raw or grilled romaine, and, of course, finished with your favorite whole-grain croutons. It's also great as a topping on sandwiches, saucing up your grains, or for dipping veggies.

½ cup raw cashews
¾ cup unsweetened plant milk
2½ tablespoons white wine vinegar
1 garlic clove
2 teaspoons sea vegetable granules, preferably nori, dulse, or wakame (avoid hijiki and kelp)
1 tablespoon natural sweetener such as fruit paste
1 tablespoon light soy or chickpea miso
1 tablespoon nutritional yeast
1½ tablespoons Dijon mustard
½ teaspoon freshly ground black pepper
Juice of ½ lemon, or more, to taste
½ teaspoon sea salt

1. In a small bowl, soak the cashews in enough warm water to cover until softened, 2 hours. Drain.

2. In blender, combine the cashews, plant milk, vinegar, garlic, kelp granules, sweetener, miso, nutritional yeast, Dijon, pepper, lemon juice, and sea salt, and blend until smooth, 5 to 10 seconds.

Note: If needed to create a smooth consistency, fold with a spatula when blending.

Peach Champagne Vinaigrette
Makes 1½ cups

RECIPE BY CHAD SARNO

This simple and fresh rustic dressing bursts with flavor; with a balance of sweet and savory herbs, it pairs perfectly with spicy greens such as arugula and even the more delicate lettuces. Swap out the peaches to high-light any seasonal fruit you wish.

½ cup muscatel vinegar or champagne vinegar
2 tablespoons apricot paste (see note)
¼ cup diced peaches
2 tablespoons finely chopped fresh chives
2 tablespoons finely chopped fresh mint
1 tablespoon grated lemon zest
¼ teaspoon freshly ground black pepper
Pinch of sea salt, or more to taste

1. In small bowl, whisk the vinegar, apricot paste, peaches, chives, mint, lemon zest, pepper, and sea salt until well-combined with a rustic, course texture.

Note: To make apricot paste, soak dried apricots in hot water for at least 1 hour. When the apricots are plump and softened, place in a blender and add enough water to cover. Blend on high to create a smooth paste. This citrusy whole food sweetener is very versatile and can be used in a variety of ways such as dressings, morning oatmeal, or desserts.

Lemon Basil Dressing   *Makes 1½ cups*

This is my daily go-to classic dressing that's super easy to customize. Substitute other fresh herbs, like dill or cilantro, or else swap out the herbs altogether for one tablespoon Dijon mustard and one teaspoon of pure maple syrup for a sweet and mild blend.

1 (15-ounce) can cannellini beans, drained and rinsed
½ cup fresh basil leaves, stems removed
3 tablespoons nutritional yeast
2 to 3 tablespoons freshly squeezed lemon juice with zest
2 tablespoons tahini
1 tablespoon tamari

1. In a blender, add the beans, ½ cup water, basil, nutritional yeast, lemon juice and zest, tahini, and tamari, and blend until smooth, 30 to 90 seconds.

2. Serve immediately or store in an airtight container in the refrigerator for 4 to 5 days.

Note: If needed to create a smooth consistency, be sure to stop the blender every 15 to 20 seconds and fold with a spatula when blending.

Cilantro Lime Dressing
Makes 1½ cups

Earthy and citrus-infused, this creamy dressing perks up any salad, baked potato, or whole grain while filling you up with a huge nutritional burst. Beans add texture along with healthy fiber while the zesty lime juice helps you absorb the iron from the cilantro and beans.

1 (15-ounce) can cannellini beans, drained and rinsed
½ cup fresh cilantro leaves
¼ cup nutritional yeast
3 tablespoons tahini
2 to 3 tablespoons tamari
2 tablespoons freshly squeezed lime juice with zest
1 tablespoon pure maple syrup
⅛ teaspoon crushed red pepper flakes

1. Using a standing blender or an immersion blender and a deep cup or jar, puree the beans, cilantro, 1/2 cup water, nutritional yeast, tahini, tamari, lime juice and zest, maple syrup, and red pepper flakes until very smooth, 30 to 90 seconds.

2. Serve immediately or store in an airtight container in the refrigerator for up to 3 or 4 days.

Note: To thin dressing, add 1 teaspoon water at a time until thinned as desired. You can make it thicker to serve as a dip by reducing the water.

Sofrito
Makes 2½ cups

Indulge in this legendary sauce of the Mediterranean, famous for its synergy in the body, and also for its delicious combination of classic flavors. Instead of olive oil, this recipe uses whole kalamata olives to contribute some fat (and delicious flavor), which enhances the absorption of the carotenoids of the tomatoes. If fresh heirloom tomatoes are available, they are divine in this recipe, but other fresh tomatoes work wonderfully as well.

6 cups chopped fresh tomatoes (preferably heirloom varieties)
1 cup chopped yellow onion
¼ cup halved Kalamata olives
2 or 3 garlic cloves, minced
2 teaspoons dried basil
1 teaspoon dried oregano
1 teaspoon dried rosemary
1 bay leaf
¼ to ½ teaspoon freshly ground black pepper
½ teaspoon salt (optional)

1. In a large pot, cover and cook the tomatoes over high heat to sweat, 5 to 10 minutes. Once tomatoes are sweating, add the onion, olives, garlic, basil, oregano, rosemary, bay leaf, black pepper, and salt. Reduce heat and cover. Simmer over low heat, stirring occasionally, until sauce thickens, 20 to 30 minutes.

2. Turn off the heat, remove the bay leaf, and puree with an immersion blender or transfer to a standing blender and puree until smooth, 10 to 20 seconds. Serve immediately over whole-grain pasta or whole grains, or use as a dip or store in an airtight container in the refrigerator for up to 4 to 5 days.

Antipasti (Small Plates)

Plural of *antipasto*, *antipasti* are traditionally the appetizer dishes served in the Mediterranean before a meal. However, in the Vegiterranean lifestyle, small plates can be eaten alone, with other small plates, for lunch, snack, or dinner, or however you desire!

Sunrise Kale Chips
Makes 2 cups

Enjoy these tangy, crunchy, zesty bites of sunrise-colored nutrition. Although these delights are slowly baked or dehydrated for several hours, they are well worth the wait. You may want to make a few batches at a time because they disappear quickly.

2 jarred roasted red bell peppers, rinsed well (about ¾ cup)
½ cup raw cashews, preferably soaked and rinsed, but not necessary
¼ cup nutritional yeast
2 tablespoons freshly squeezed lemon juice with zest
1 tablespoon tahini
2 teaspoons tamari or Bragg liquid aminos
¼ teaspoon crushed red pepper flakes
1 bunch curly kale, de-stemmed and torn into pieces

1. Preheat the oven to 170°F. Line 2 baking sheets with silicone liners or parchment paper.

2. In a blender, add the bell peppers, cashews, nutritional yeast, lemon juice and zest, tahini, tamari, and red pepper flakes, and blend on high speed until well-combined, 30 to 60 seconds.

3. Place the kale in a large bowl and pour the bell pepper sauce evenly over the kale, massaging the sauce into the leaves with your hands, until thoroughly distributed. Uniformly space out the kale on the prepared baking sheets, allowing for space in between the leaves.

4. Bake until kale is crispy and completely dry, 3 1/2 to 4 hours, stirring the kale every hour with tongs or a spatula, rearranging as evenly as possible before returning to the oven each time. Or if you have a dehydrator, dehydrate on medium (about 125° F) for approximately 6 to 8 hours.

5. Serve immediately or place in an airtight container in refrigerator for up to 4 or 5 days.

Easy Caprese   *Makes 2 to 4 servings*

A simple, traditional dish, this combination satisfies as a perfect appetizer. Hearty in texture, but zesty and light in flavor, you can throw this together in minutes and enjoy as a light snack in the afternoon or before dinner.

2 large heirloom or beefsteak tomatoes, sliced into ½-inch-thick slices
⅓ cup fresh basil leaves

4 ounces organic soft tofu, thinly sliced
2 to 3 tablespoons reduced balsamic vinegar

1. Layer the tomato slices on a large plate. Evenly place the basil leaves over the tomatoes, followed by the tofu slices. Drizzle the vinegar over all.

2. Serve immediately or store in an airtight container in the refrigerator for up to 2 days.

Note: You can use your favorite regular balsamic vinegar as is, or try reducing it. Using at least triple the amount of vinegar called for in the recipe in a saucepan (you can store the leftovers in the refrigerator for up to a week), bring the vinegar to a boil over medium heat, and then reduce the heat to low and simmer until at desired thickness, at least 20 to 30 minutes.

Potato Cups *Makes 6 to 8 servings*

Inspired by the creative Chloe Coscarelli's Mini Potato Skins in her first book, *Chloe's Kitchen,* I discovered that using potatoes as edible vessels for a number of different ingredients make the perfect appetizer, snack, or even a meal. They are always a huge hit at parties, and you can stuff them with your favorite filling. My favorites combine hummus with salsa, guacamole with salsa, or just one of those three alone.

10 to 12 small or 6 to 8 medium new potatoes or Yukon gold potatoes
2 cups filling of choice

1. Preheat the oven to 375°F.

2. Place the whole potatoes on a baking sheet lined with a silicone liner or parchment paper. Bake until mostly cooked through, 20 to 30 minutes. Set aside the potatoes to cool, but do not turn off the oven.

3. Once cooled, slice the potatoes in half. With a melon baller, scoop out a hole in each half. (Reserve potato pulp for soup or to make mashed potatoes.)

4. Return the potato cup to the oven and bake until slightly browned on top, 10 to 15 minutes. Fill the potato hollows with your choice of

hummus, salsa, guacamole, chili, beans, or other desired filling. Serve hot. These will store well in airtight containers in the refrigerator for 3 to 4 days as long as they are not filled.

Lemon Chard with Chickpeas   *Makes 2 to 4 servings*

Sour, spicy, and tangy, this dish is the perfect way to bring in the greens! The vitamin C helps you absorb the iron in the chard and chickpeas and makes this a delicious synergistic combination you'll want to eat regularly.

    1 to 4 garlic cloves, minced
    ¼ cup vegetable stock
    1 bunch Swiss chard, chopped (about 4 leaves)
    1 (15-ounce) can chickpeas
    1 tablespoon turmeric
    1 tablespoon ground cumin
    1 tablespoon sweet paprika
    1½ tablespoons freshly squeezed lemon juice
    ½ cup crushed tomatoes
    1 cup water or vegetable stock

1. In a large pot, saute the garlic in ¼ cup vegetable stock over medium-high heat just until softened, 1 to 2 minutes. (Do not allow garlic to brown.) Add the chard and cook, stirring occasionally, until beginning to wilt, 2 minutes.

2. Toss in the chickpeas, turmeric, cumin, paprika, lemon juice, tomatoes, and 1 cup water, and bring to a boil. Once boiling, reduce heat and simmer until the greens are softened, 10 to 15 minutes. Serve warm with rice, if desired. Serve immediately or store in an airtight container in the refrigerator for up to 2 to 3 days.

Dilled Rice with Lima Beans   *Makes 2 to 4 servings*

My dearest friend, Donna, makes the best Persian rice, and she always includes it on the menu when I come for dinner. This recipe uses the same delicious flavor combinations of turmeric and dill, but omits the oil for a lower-calorie, but flavor-filled version. Enjoy this as a main dish, as an addition over salad, or paired with a main dish, such as Green *Ful*, *Ful Medames*, or Hearty Red Lentil Stew.

1 cup dry, brown basmati rice
2 teaspoons turmeric
1 cup frozen lima beans, thawed
¼ cup finely chopped fresh dill
Pinch of salt and freshly ground black pepper, or more to taste

1. In a medium pot, combine the rice, turmeric, and 3 cups water, and bring to a boil over high heat. Once boiling, reduce heat; cover and simmer, stirring occasionally to avoid sticking, until most of the water is absorbed and the rice is cooked, 30 to 35 minutes.

2. Add lima beans and 1 cup water. Cover and simmer until beans are cooked through, 5 to 7 minutes. Add dill, salt, and pepper and stir. Cover and simmer to heat through, 1 minute. Turn off heat and keep covered until ready to serve.

3. Serve immediately or store in an airtight container in the refrigerator for up to 5 to 6 days.

Simple Roasted Vegetables   *Makes 2 to 4 servings*

Roasting vegetables brings out their natural sugars, making them sweeter and more flavorful. Traditionally, this is an essential side dish for large spreads or can be enjoyed on their own with minimal preparation. Served over cooked whole grains these veggies become a full meal.

1 large eggplant, sliced into ½-inch rounds
½ large red bell pepper, seeded and sliced into thick slices (about 4)
1 medium yellow zucchini, sliced diagonally into ½-inch pieces
1 medium green zucchini, sliced diagonally into ½-inch pieces
½ teaspoon salt (optional)
1 teaspoon freshly ground black pepper
2 tablespoons chopped fresh basil, stems removed
3 to 4 tablespoons balsamic vinegar (preferably reduced)

1. Preheat the oven to 375°F.

2. On a baking sheet lined with a silicone liner or parchment paper, place the eggplant, bell pepper, yellow zucchini, and green zucchini. Sprinkle with the salt and pepper.

3. Roast until browned, 15 minutes. Turn all the vegetables over and roast until browned, 10 more minutes. Remove from the oven and place on a dish. Sprinkle the basil and vinegar evenly over the vegetables and serve immediately or store in an airtight container in the refrigerator for up to 2 to 3 days.

Delicious Dolmas
Makes 6 to 8 servings

A classic in the family of traditionally stuffed vegetables served in Greece, Turkey, and the Middle East, grape leaves serve as a wrapper to hold a filling of rice, dried fruits, and seasonings. Garlic, mint, and lemon infuse the dolmas as they cook in the oven. Although this dish requires time and patience, it is awe-inspiring.

1 (16-ounce) jar grape leaves, rinsed well
1 cup finely chopped yellow onion
2¾ cups vegetable stock, divided
4 cups cooked brown rice
2 tablespoons minced fresh basil
6 medium-size pitted dates, finely chopped
6 dried apricots, finely chopped
¼ cup finely chopped raisins
1 garlic clove, minced
1 teaspoon ground cumin
2 teaspoons turmeric, divided
1½ teaspoons freshly ground black pepper, divided
Pinch of salt (optional)
10 grape tomatoes, halved, divided
3 large garlic cloves, sliced into 6 pieces, divided
8 fresh mint leaves, divided
1 tablespoon freshly squeezed lemon juice
¼ teaspoon crushed red pepper flakes

1. Rinse the grape leaves (however many you plan on eating) from the jar in a colander with plenty of water to remove the salt. Set aside.

2. In a medium pan, saute the onion in 3/4 cup vegetable stock over medium heat until onion is translucent, 5 minutes. Add the rice and turn off the heat. Mix in the basil, dates, apricots, raisins, garlic, cumin, 1 teaspoon turmeric, 1 teaspoon pepper, and salt, and stir to combine.

3. Preheat oven to 350°F.

4. On a flat, clean surface, spread out the grape leaves, one at a time. Place a small scoop of the rice mixture in the center, bottom of the leaf. Tuck the sides in and roll up to make cigar-shaped rolls, wrapping as tightly as possible.

5. In a deep, oval-shaped 8 x 8-inch casserole dish, place the stuffed Dolmas in one layer (approximately 18) to cover the bottom of the dish. On top of the first layer, place 10 grape tomatoes halves, 18 garlic slices, and 4 mint leaves.

6. Next, layer another 18 stuffed Dolmas on top and cover with 10 grape tomato halves, 18 garlic slices, and 4 mint leaves. Drizzle the lemon juice evenly over all.

7. In a small bowl, combine 2 cups vegetable stock, 1/4 cup water, 1 teaspoon turmeric, 1/2 teaspoon pepper, and red pepper flakes. Pour over the stuffed Dolmas evenly. Cover and bake until slightly swollen, 30 minutes. Serve immediately or store in an airtight container in the refrigerator for up to 5 to 6 days.

Note: Grape leaf sizes vary so try to maintain consistency among the sizes used and the amount of filling as best as possible to promote even cooking.

Rainbow Stuffed Cabbage Rolls   *Makes 6 to 8 servings*

A traditional dish in the Middle East, these fragrant dumplings are bursting with just the right amount of sweet and savory. Omitting the customary animal products and hefty dose of oil make these healthful and light, providing a rainbow on your plate of excellent, pure nourishment. Although time-consuming with intricate preparation required, these delicacies are well worth the effort. Save these to serve at holidays and special occasions to share with family and friends.

¼ cup chopped dried apricots
2 cups boiling water
1 large head green cabbage
½ large yellow onion, grated
1 large carrot, grated
1 large zucchini, grated
2 cups cooked brown rice
¼ cup chopped fresh dill
2 tablespoons chopped fresh parsley
¼ cup golden raisins
1 garlic clove, minced
1 tablespoon plus ½ teaspoon turmeric, divided
1 tablespoon plus ½ teaspoon ground cumin, divided
1 tablespoon plus ½ teaspoon sweet paprika, divided
1½ teaspoons freshly ground black pepper, divided
2 tablespoons freshly squeezed lemon juice, divided
1 cup crushed tomatoes
½ teaspoon salt (optional)

1. In a small bowl, soak the dried apricots in the boiling water, setting aside.

2. Place the cabbage head on its top with the core right side up. Using a large knife, slice 4 punctures into the cabbage head around the periphery of the core to help facilitate leaf separation later.

3. In a large 3- or 4-quart pot filled three-quarters of the way with water, bring the water to a boil over medium-high heat. Once boiling, place the cabbage head into the pot with the core right side up, and cook until the outer cabbage leaves are softened, 5 minutes. Every 3 to 5 minutes, remove the cabbage with 2 forks on either side, bring to a colander in the sink, and peel off the outermost layer. Return the remaining cabbage head to the boiling water and repeat until you have 15 to 20 separated cabbage leaves. Set aside.

4. To make the filling, place the onion, carrot, zucchini, brown rice, dill, parsley, raisins, garlic, 1 tablespoon turmeric, 1 tablespoon cumin, 1 tablespoon paprika, 1 teaspoon black pepper, and 1 tablespoon lemon juice in a medium bowl. Toss to combine.

5. Remove the dried apricots from the soaking water, reserving 1 cup of the soaking water for the sauce. Prepare a deep 6-quart casserole dish by placing a layer of one-half of the soaked apricots on the bottom.

6. Preheat the oven to 350°F.

7. On a flat surface, remove the stem from 1 cabbage leaf, cutting in half if large. Place 1 teaspoon filling onto the bottom center portion of the leaf. Fold the bottom over the filling, grabbing with your fingers, and then fold the sides in and roll the remaining leaf to look like a tiny burrito. Place in the baking dish, starting a layer on top of the apricots. Repeat with a layer of the remaining apricots and then a layer of the remaining cabbage leaves and filling, covering the apricots with the cabbage rolls. (You should fill about 20 to 25 cabbage rolls.)

8. Combine the tomatoes, reserved apricot soaking water, ½ teaspoon turmeric, ½ teaspoon cumin, ½ teaspoon paprika, ½ teaspoon black pepper, 1 tablespoon lemon juice, and salt in a small bowl. Pour over the stuffed cabbages, distributing evenly. Cover and bake until browned on top, 40 minutes. Serve hot or store in an airtight container in the refrigerator for up to 4 to 5 days.

Insalata e Zuppe (Salads and Soups)

Salads are by definition any combination of ready-to-eat raw and/or cooked vegetables and commonly served with a dressing. They can range from simple to abundant, including heartier ingredients to make a satisfying meal. Soups are not limited with their ingredients; they can be light and brothy or thicker, such as a chowder. Because both raw and cooked vegetables are important for a healthy diet, salads and soups are excellent to include at least once per day. Soups maintain much of the nutrients lost when cooking because the liquid is consumed so they are an excellent way of including water-sensitive minerals and vitamins.

Breakfast Sunshine Salad   *Makes 2 to 4 servings*

Yes, salad for breakfast! Bring fresh to your morning with this crunchy and simple dish. Infused with sweetness and zest, you can throw this together in five minutes, and it is a great way to start your day with all of those fruits and veggies. This would also make a great dessert.

3 or 4 medium-size carrots, shredded (2 cups)
½ cup raisins or currants
2 tablespoons unsweetened shredded coconut
1 banana, cut into disks (1 cup)
1 orange, halved, divided

1. In a medium bowl, combine the carrots, raisins, coconut, and banana. Squeeze the juice from half of the orange over the salad, and stir to combine.

2. Chop up the remaining half of the orange into small pieces and add to the salad. Serve immediately or store in an airtight container in the refrigerator for 2 to 3 days.

Israeli Salad

Makes 1 to 4 servings

A basic, crisp, always welcoming side dish, this salad is a necessity in the Middle East (on the Med). Eat it with every meal and adjust according to your preferences. Fresh herbs, such as basil, cilantro, parsley, and dill, provide an additional infused essence.

1 cup chopped unpeeled cucumber
1 cup chopped tomato
½ cup chopped red bell pepper
1 tablespoon chopped fresh cilantro
1 tablespoon chopped fresh Italian flat-leaf parsley
2 tablespoons freshly squeezed lemon juice with zest
Pinch of salt (optional)
½ teaspoon minced jalapeno pepper (optional)

1. Combine the cucumber, tomato, bell pepper, cilantro, and parsley in a medium bowl.

2. Pour the lemon juice and zest over top, and add salt and jalapeño. Toss to combine and serve immediately. It will keep in an airtight con-

tainer stored in the refrigerator for up to 2 days, but fresh is best, as it loses its crispness rapidly.

Tabbouleh
Makes 2 to 4 servings

This traditional Arabic dish can be made with quinoa for a gluten-free version (see Quinoa and Chickpea Tabbouleh Salad). Bulgur is a nutty-flavored cracked wheat that pleasantly contrasts with the fresh, crisp vegetables and aromatics. This salad can be served with hummus and pita or over romaine lettuce for a main dish.

> 1 cup uncooked bulgur
> ½ medium red onion, thinly sliced
> 1½ cups seeded, finely chopped unpeeled cucumber
> 1 cup chopped tomatoes
> ½ cup minced fresh mint
> 2 tablespoons minced fresh Italian flat-leaf parsley
> 2 to 3 tablespoons freshly squeezed lemon juice with zest
> ½ teaspoon freshly ground black pepper
> ¼ teaspoon salt

1. Soak the bulgur in enough water to cover until softened, 1 hour. Drain well.

2. In a medium bowl, combine the bulgur, onion, cucumber, tomatoes, mint, and parsley. Toss to combine. Add the lemon juice and zest and sprinkle with pepper and salt. Toss again.

3. Serve immediately or store in an airtight container in the refrigerator for up to 4 days.

Quinoa and Chickpea Tabbouleh Salad
Makes 4 servings

Light and herb-infused, this salad is refreshing and extremely nutritious. Traditionally made with bulgur wheat, this gluten-free version boasts similar flavors, but it's friendly for those eschewing gluten and more substantial because of the added chickpeas.

3 to 4 tablespoons freshly squeezed lemon juice with zest
½ teaspoon freshly ground black pepper
½ teaspoon salt (optional)
1 garlic clove, minced (optional)
2 cups cooked quinoa
1 (15-ounce) can chickpeas, rinsed and drained
1 large unpeeled cucumber, seeded and diced
¾ cup halved grape or cherry tomatoes
¾ cup finely chopped Italian flat-leaf parsley
¾ cup finely chopped fresh mint leaves
¼ cup chopped finely scallions

1. In a medium bowl, whisk together the lemon juice and zest, pepper, salt, and garlic. Fold in the quinoa, chickpeas, cucumber, tomatoes, parsley, mint, and scallions, and combine well.

2. Serve immediately, or cover and refrigerate. Serve cold or at room temperature. Store leftovers in an airtight container in the refrigerator for up to 4 days.

Tuscan Garden Salad with Fresh Tomato Dressing

Makes 4 servings

RECIPE BY ROBIN ROBERTSON

The dressing for this salad is so delicious you may want to drink it, but save some for the salad featuring creamy chickpeas, crisp vegetables, and luscious Kalamata olives.

DRESSING
1 large ripe tomato, cored, seeded, and coarsely chopped
1 tablespoon rice vinegar
1 small garlic clove, crushed
1 small pitted date
2 teaspoons nutritional yeast
¼ teaspoon sea salt
⅛ teaspoon dried oregano
⅛ teaspoon freshly ground black pepper

SALAD
1 large head romaine lettuce, chopped
1½ cups cooked or 1 (15-ounce) can chickpeas, drained and rinsed
1½ cups halved grape or cherry tomatoes
½ small unpeeled cucumber, thinly sliced
½ yellow bell pepper, diced
¼ cup small basil leaves
2 tablespoons Kalamata olives, pitted and halved

1. To make the dressing, combine the tomato, vinegar, 1 tablespoon water, garlic, date, nutritional yeast, salt, oregano, and pepper in a high-speed blender. Blend until smooth, 10 to 20 seconds. If not using right away, transfer the dressing to a jar or other container with a tight-fitting lid and refrigerate until needed. Properly stored, the dressing will keep for 2 to 3 days.

2. To make the salad, combine the lettuce, chickpeas, tomatoes, cucumber, bell pepper, basil, and olives in a large bowl. Add the dressing and toss to coat. Serve immediately.

Red Hot Eggplant Salad

Makes 1½ cups

Hot salads bring a whole new opportunity for vegetable creativity. This warm and spicy salad makes a great side dish or addition to a cold green salad. This hot combo is exploding with antioxidants and phytochemicals galore thanks to the spices and cooked carotenoid-dense veggies.

½ large unpeeled eggplant, cubed
½ large yellow onion, chopped
½ red bell pepper, chopped
1 cup crushed tomatoes
3 garlic cloves, minced
1 tablespoon crushed red pepper flakes
1 tablespoon turmeric
1 teaspoon ground cumin
½ teaspoon salt (optional)

1. Preheat oven to 400°F.

2. On a baking sheet lined with a silicone liner or parchment paper, place the eggplant, onion, and red bell pepper separately. Bake until browned, 30 minutes. Remove the vegetables from the oven and transfer to a small pot.

3. Add tomatoes, ¼ cup water, garlic, red pepper flakes, turmeric, cumin, and salt. Bring to a boil over medium-high heat. Once boiling, reduce heat to low and cook, stirring occasionally, until most of the sauce is absorbed, 15 to 20 minutes.

4. Serve hot or refrigerate and serve cold with pita bread or as a condiment. Try serving it in a whole-grain pita bread with tahini. It will store in an airtight container in the refrigerator for up to 4 to 5 days.

Hot, Sweet, and Sour Bhamia (Okra)

Makes 4 to 6 servings

Okra, known as *bhamia* in the Middle East, is an edible green seedpod vegetable enjoyed widely around the Mediterranean. Many people tend to dislike okra because of its gummy consistency; cooking with acidic ingredients such as tomato or lemon juice softens its unique consistency while infusing it with flavor.

1 cup chopped yellow onion
1½ cups vegetable stock, divided
1 cup red bell pepper, seeded and sliced into 4 pieces
1 Yukon gold potato, peeled and halved
1 (12-ounce) package frozen okra
2 garlic cloves, minced
2 dried apricots
1 tablespoon turmeric
1 teaspoon cumin
½ teaspoon freshly ground black pepper
½ teaspoon crushed red pepper flakes
½ teaspoon salt (optional)
1 cup crushed tomatoes
1 tablespoon freshly squeezed lemon juice with zest

1. In a medium pot, saute the onion in ½ cup vegetable stock over medium heat until translucent, 5 minutes. Add bell pepper, potato, frozen okra, garlic, apricots, turmeric, cumin, pepper, crushed red pepper flakes, and salt. Cook over low heat until vegetables soften, 5 minutes.

2. Add tomatoes and 1 cup vegetable stock and bring to a boil. Once boiling, reduce heat to medium-low. Cover and simmer until half of the sauce is absorbed, 10 minutes. Add lemon juice and zest and cook until heated through, 5 minutes. Serve immediately over rice, if desired, or store in an airtight container in the refrigerator for up to 3 to 4 days.

Couscous Soup
Makes 6 to 8 servings

Couscous is a traditional grain used in the Mediterranean, made of semolina and granules of durum wheat. Served in a soup, couscous complements the vegetables, making it more of a robust stew.

  1 medium-size yellow onion, diced
  4 cups vegetable stock, divided
  4 large carrots, chopped in large chunks
  3 ribs celery, chopped in large chunks
  2 cups chopped butternut squash
  1 (15-ounce) can chickpeas, drained and rinsed
  5 medium-size potatoes, peeled and chopped
  ½ cup chopped fresh dill
  2 teaspoons turmeric
  1 teaspoon ground cumin
  1 teaspoon crushed red pepper flakes
  ½ teaspoon salt (optional)
  1 (10-ounce) package couscous

1. In a medium soup pot, saute the onion in ½ cup vegetable stock over medium-high heat until the onion is translucent, 5 minutes. Add carrots, celery, squash, and chickpeas, and cook until the vegetables are soft, 5 to 10 minutes.

2. Add potatoes, dill, 3½ cups vegetable stock, 6 cups water, turmeric, cumin, red pepper flakes, and salt. Bring to a boil over medium-high heat.

Once boiling, reduce heat and simmer over medium heat until the potatoes are tender, for 30 minutes.

3. Meanwhile, in a small pot over medium-high heat, bring 2 cups water to a boil. Once boiling, pour in the couscous, turn off the heat, and cover. Let stand until all liquid is absorbed, 10 to 15 minutes. Fluff with a fork.

4. Serve immediately by placing some couscous in a bowl and topping with the soup or store soup and couscous separately in airtight containers in the refrigerator for up to 4 days.

Hatz Lentil Soup

Makes 4 to 6 servings

This red lentil soup made in Alexandria, Egypt, traditionally is made on a cold, rainy day to warm and soothe. While the soup is simmering and the separate spice mixture is boiling, combining the two while hot is believed to bring out the earthy, piquant, and succulent flavors.

1 cup chopped yellow onion
4½ cups vegetable stock, divided
2 cups red lentils, rinsed
3 garlic cloves, minced
2 tablespoons ground cumin
1 tablespoon turmeric
1 tablespoon crushed red pepper flakes
1 teaspoon freshly ground black pepper
½ teaspoon salt (optional)

1. In a medium soup pot, saute the onion in ¼ cup vegetable stock over medium-high heat until the onion is translucent, 5 minutes. Add the lentils, 4 cups vegetable stock, 4 cups water, and bring to a boil. Once boiling, reduce heat, cover, and simmer over medium heat until lentils are soft and mushy, 30 minutes.

2. In a separate saucepan, place ¼ cup vegetable stock, garlic, cumin, turmeric, red pepper flakes, pepper, and salt. Over medium-high heat, bring to a boil. Once boiling, pour directly into the simmering soup and stir to combine.

3. Serve hot with toasted whole-grain bread, if desired, or store in an airtight container in the refrigerator for up to 4 to 5 days.

Potato Corn Chowder   *Makes 2 to 4 servings*

Potatoes were a staple in Crete during the time of the studies, especially in the rural areas. Starchy vegetables have always provided accessible, nutrient-dense sustenance in a culinary-ily versatile and delicious way. This comforting and creamy soup is the perfectly soothing pick-me-up. Lightly seasoned, it is hearty and wonderfully satisfying.

1 medium yellow onion, diced
4 cups vegetable stock, divided
1 green bell pepper, chopped
2 ribs celery, chopped
2 cups frozen corn
2 medium-size Russet potatoes, peeled and chopped
1 bay leaf
1 teaspoon freshly ground black pepper
2 tablespoons chopped fresh dill
2 cups plain, unsweetened plant milk

1. In a medium soup pot, saute the onion in ½ cup vegetable stock over medium-high heat until onion is translucent, 5 minutes. Add the bell pepper, celery, and corn, and cook until vegetables soften, 5 more minutes.

2. Add the potatoes, 3½ cups vegetable stock, bay leaf, pepper, and dill. Bring to a boil. Once boiling, reduce heat and simmer over medium heat until the vegetables are soft, 15 to 20 minutes.

3. Pour in the plant milk and increase heat, bringing the soup to a boil. Reduce heat and cook over low heat until vegetables soften, an additional 5 minutes.

4. Turn off heat and remove bay leaf. With an immersion blender, puree the soup until most is pureed, but some remains chunky. Cook until thickened, 5 to 10 more minutes. Serve hot with whole-grain bread, if desired, or store in an airtight container in the refrigerator for up to 4 to 6 days.

Pane e Panini (Breads and Sandwiches)

Warm bread was the crux of the diet in post World War II Crete, as well as in the Mediterranean. Of course, bread is still enjoyed around much of the Western world, as an appetizer; for sandwiches; and served with soups, dips, and main dishes. Made wholesome with intact grains, bread is a versatile staple we can relish healthfully in the Vegiterranean diet.

Baked Oat Bread   *Makes 1 loaf*

Eating Vegiterranean would be incomplete without a staple whole-grain bread to add to a meal. This bread is gluten-free, soft, and guilt-free. Baking bread is the ultimate in science meeting art so follow the directions carefully, make sure the yeast is fresh, and be sure you begin preparation several hours ahead of mealtime.

1½ teaspoons active dry yeast
2 tablespoons pure maple syrup
2 cups warm (not hot) water
3½ cups oat flour
1¾ teaspoons salt
2 tablespoons hemp, poppy, pumpkin, sesame, or sunflower seeds
   (optional)

1. In a large bowl, combine the yeast, maple syrup, and warm water. Stir gently with your fingers, cover with plastic wrap, and set aside until bubbles rise to the top, about 10 minutes.

2. Once the yeast become active, pour in oat flour, 1 cup at a time, stirring well. Add salt and stir until well combined. Cover with plastic wrap and let stand in a dry, warm area for at least 90 minutes.

3. When the dough appears puffy and has risen, push it down, using the plastic wrap (it is very sticky) and cover again.

4. Preheat the oven to 350°F.

5. Transfer the dough to a 9 x 5-inch silicon loaf pan and shape evenly throughout. Sprinkle the seeds over the top and press gently into dough.

Bake until the bread appears lightly browned on edges, 20 minutes. Do not overcook.

6. Allow the bread to cool in the pan. Serve immediately or store in the refrigerator for up to 3 or 4 days. Toast before serving, if refrigerated.

Stone-Ground Cornbread   *Makes 6 to 8 servings*

Whole cornmeal is frequently used in traditionally rustic Mediterranean breads. This is a basic bread with a subtle sweetness plus a hint of heat that pairs nicely with a stew or chili or tastes delicious on its own as a breakfast bread.

1½ tablespoons ground flaxseed
1 cup plain, unsweetened almond (or other plant) milk
½ cup applesauce
½ cup pure maple syrup
1 cup cornmeal
1 cup oat flour
1 teaspoon baking powder
1 teaspoon baking soda
½ teaspoon salt
1 cup frozen fire-roasted or plain corn kernels, thawed, or canned corn, drained
1 tablespoon canned diced green chilies (optional)

1. Preheat the oven to 350°F.

2. In a small mixing bowl, combine the flaxseed with the almond milk, and set aside to gel for a few minutes. Add the applesauce and maple syrup, and stir to combine.

3. In a separate bowl, place the cornmeal, oat flour, baking powder, baking soda, and salt, and whisk to combine. Add the wet ingredients to the dry ingredients, and combine well, but without overmixing. Once well incorporated, stir in the corn and chilies.

4. Pour the batter into a 9 x 5-inch loaf pan. Bake until lightly browned on top and a toothpick or knife comes out clean, 30 to 35 minutes. Allow to cool in pan. Serve immediately or store in the refrigerator for up to 3 or 4 days. Toast before serving, if refrigerated.

Carrot Muffins

Makes 12 muffins

Nothing like a lightly sweet, soft, and satisfying way to add more bright, colorful vegetables into your day. Enjoy these whole-grain treats on their own, with a meal, or just as dessert.

1½ tablespoons ground flaxseed
1 cup unsweetened almond milk
½ cup unsweetened applesauce
½ cup pure maple syrup
2 cups oat flour
1 teaspoon baking powder
1 teaspoon baking soda
½ teaspoon salt
1 teaspoon ground cinnamon
½ teaspoon ground nutmeg
¼ teaspoon ground ginger
1 cup shredded carrots

1. Preheat the oven to 350°F.

2. In a small bowl, combine the flaxseed, almond milk, applesauce, and maple syrup. Stir and set aside.

3. In a large bowl, combine the oat flour, baking powder, baking soda, salt, cinnamon, nutmeg, and ginger, and mix well.

4. Add the wet mixture to the dry mixture, gently folding and mixing until just combined. (Be careful not to overmix.) Fold in the carrots.

5. Spoon the batter into a 12-cup silicon muffin pan or other lined muffin pan. Bake until muffins are lightly browned and toothpick inserted into center comes out clean, 25 to 30 minutes.

6. Allow to cool, and then transfer muffins to a cooling rack. Serve immediately or store in the refrigerator for up to 3 days.

Banana Sandwich

Makes 1 sandwich

Mom is happy because of the banana, nut butter, and hempseeds; chocolate chips serve as the bribe to make the kids crave this yummy treat. A perfectly delicious compromise for breakfast, snack, or dessert!

1 banana
1 tablespoon nut or seed butter
1 to 2 teaspoons hempseeds
8 dark, dairy-free chocolate chips (grain-sweetened, if possible)

1. On a flat surface, slice banana in half, widthwise. Then, carefully slice the 2 pieces lengthwise so you have 4 pieces. On the inside of one half of each pair, spread the nut butter evenly. Sprinkle with hempseeds and plant 4 chocolate chips per side. Close up the sandwich and enjoy.

Savory Veggie Pancakes   *Makes 2 to 4 servings*

Instead of the standard sweet breakfast pancake, shake up the usual and have pancakes for dinner. These pancakes are filled with protein and are so satisfying. Have fun experimenting with different types of vegetables, just shred or chop them finely. Top with a dressing, hummus, sauce, or even use them as a bread to dip with.

½ cup shredded carrots
¼ cup shredded or finely chopped red or other bell pepper
¼ cup shredded or finely chopped yellow onion
1 tablespoon chopped fresh Italian flat-leaf parsley
¼ to ½ teaspoon freshly ground black pepper
1 cup chickpea flour
½ teaspoon baking powder
¼ to ½ teaspoon salt

1. In a medium bowl, combine the carrots, bell pepper, onion, parsley, and pepper. Whisk in chickpea flour, baking powder, and salt. Then slowly add 1 cup water, breaking up lumps.

2. Heat a medium pan over medium-high heat. Once hot, using a ladle, scoop in some of the batter to make medium-size pancakes. Cook until bubbles form on the edges and center, 1 to 2 minutes. Flip the pancake and cook to lightly brown the other side, 1 to 2 minutes. Repeat until all the batter is used. Serve immediately for best results or store in an airtight container in the refrigerator for up to 3 to 4 days.

Roasted Vegetable Sandwich Rolls   *Makes 4 to 6 servings*

A warm, toasty panini with sweet vegetables and a clever twist is perfect in the winter when served with soup. This dish, brilliantly constructed by Miri, is slightly extraordinary with its roulade twist, an ode to warm, toasty, wrap-like sandwiches.

> 1 large eggplant, sliced into ½-inch rounds
> 1 large red bell pepper, seeded and sliced into thick slices (about 8)
> ½ teaspoon salt
> 1 teaspoon freshly ground black pepper
> 1 large French bread loaf
> ¾ cup Betta' than Feta cheese (See page 183 for recipe.)

1. Preheat the oven to 375°F.

2. On a baking sheet covered with a silicone liner or parchment paper, place the eggplant and bell pepper slices. Sprinkle with the salt and pepper. Roast until browned, 15 minutes. Flip the vegetables and bake until browned on the other side,10 more minutes.

3. On a dry, flat surface, cut the French bread loaf lengthwise halfway through, keeping one half together. Remove the bread from inside, leaving only the outer crust. Place the roasted eggplant and bell peppers into the loaf and cover with Betta' than Feta.

4. Start from one of the wide sides and tightly roll the entire sandwich into a roulade. Wrap aluminum foil with parchment paper (parchment paper is in direct contact with the food) around the roulade. Bake until the bread is toasted, 8 to 10 minutes.

5. Slice the sandwich into 3-inch slices. Serve warm with Baba Ganoush (see page 192), Tahina (see page 191), and/or hummus, if desired. This is best served immediately, but ingredients can be stored in the refrigerator without the bread for up to 3 to 4 days and then the sandwich can be assembled when ready to eat.

Tempeh Cutlet Sandwich with Arugula and Basil Aioli

Makes 5 sandwiches

RECIPE BY CHAD SARNO

This Italian-inspired plant-based sandwich is the perfect fit to your menu when you are looking for that comfort meal. Tempeh is best prepared by braising or steaming before using to help cut the bitterness that some varieties may carry and to add moisture to this versatile plant-based protein. These savory, crusted cutlets are complemented with a generous amount of egg-free aioli.

TEMPEH CUTLETS
4 cups vegetable stock
1 cup dry white wine
1 bay leaf
¼ cup wheat-free tamari
2 tablespoons maple syrup
2 sprigs fresh rosemary
2 (8-ounce) packs tempeh

BREADING
½ cup all-purpose gluten-free flour
¼ cup nutritional yeast
1½ tablespoons onion granules
1 tablespoon garlic granules
2 tablespoons minced chives
1 tablespoon minced rosemary
1 teaspoon sea salt

SANDWICHES
10 slices whole-grain or gluten-free bread or 5 large tortillas
1½ cups baby arugula
1 small red onion, sliced paper thin
2 vine-ripened tomatoes, sliced
½ cup Basil Aioli (recipe follows)

1. To prepare the braising liquid for the tempeh cutlets, place a small pot over medium heat. Pour in the vegetable stock, wine, bay leaf, tamari,

maple syrup, and rosemary, and bring to a simmer. Be sure not to boil, keeping the braising liquid at an even simmer.

2. Slice the tempeh, on the bias, into 6 to 8 thin slices for each tempeh block. Place gently into the simmering braising liquid and cook until browned, 30 minutes. Remove from heat and keep tempeh in liquid while you prepare the breading.

3. Preheat the oven to 375°F.

4. For breading, hand-mix the flour, nutritional yeast, onion granules, garlic granules, chives, rosemary, and salt well in a small bowl. Set up a breading station by having the cooked tempeh in braising liquid, breading mixture, and a plate or rack to place the cutlets once dredged. For each piece of tempeh, remove from the liquid and place in the breading bowl, patting and coating each side. Set on a separate plate or rack. Follow this process until all tempeh pieces are breaded.

5. Place the breaded tempeh on a silicon baking pan and bake until golden brown, 10 minutes. Flip each piece and bake until cutlets are crisp, 6 to 8 minutes.

6. To assemble the tempeh sandwiches, layer the tempeh, arugula, onion, and tomato on 5 bread slices. Spread Basil Aioli onto the remaining 5 bread slices and close sandwiches. Serve immediately.

Basil Aioli

Makes 2 cups

Use this aioli as the base for a creamy, dairy-free dressing, a dollop to finish grilled or roasted vegetables, or as a savory spread on sandwiches, wraps, or crostini.

1½ cups raw cashews
Juice and zest of ½ lemon
1 garlic clove
2 tablespoons cider vinegar
½ teaspoon sea salt
2 tablespoons minced shallots
½ cup loosely packed basil

1. Soak the cashews in enough warm water to cover until softened, 2 hours. Drain.

2. In a high-speed blender, combine the cashews, ¼ cup water, lemon juice, garlic, vinegar, and sea salt. Blend, folding as necessary with a rubber spatula to ensure a smooth consistency, until smooth, 10 to 20 seconds.

3. Pour the cashew mixture into a bowl and hand-mix in the lemon zest and shallots. Mince the basil and fold into the aioli. Serve immediately or store in an airtight container in the refrigerator for up to 3 days.

Piatti Principali (Main Dishes)

Main dishes come in all styles and preferences. You may enjoy having one center of the dish or, instead, include a dollop of several options at once, smorgasbord style. Again, there is no right or wrong way to eat, so long as you are happy. Light breakfast "main dishes" are included here, as well as day- and evening-type meals such as stews, a falafel recipe, and more. Make them mains or sides, based on personal inclination.

Belila
Makes 2 to 4 servings

In Egypt, this warm cereal is served as breakfast, made from cooked wheat, warm milk, and sugar, with added nuts, raisins, shredded coconut, cinnamon, cardamom, or other flavors. Here is a healthified gluten-free, plant-based version that cooks quickly because it uses quinoa. Add any of your favorite toppings, such as fresh, frozen, or dried fruits, seeds, or different spices to this basic recipe.

    1 cup quinoa, rinsed
    1 cup unsweetened plant milk
    2 tablespoons pure maple syrup
    2 tablespoons chopped nuts (optional)
    ½ teaspoon cinnamon
    ⅛ teaspoon cardamom (optional)

1. In a medium pot, bring 2½ cups water and quinoa to a boil. Reduce heat, cover, and simmer over medium-low heat until water is absorbed, 15 minutes.

2. Fluff quinoa with a fork and add the milk, maple syrup, nuts, cinnamon, and cardamom. Cook over low heat until milk is heated, 3 to 5 minutes. Serve warm with fresh fruit on top, if desired, or store in an airtight container in the refrigerator for up to 3 to 4 days.

Shakshuka (Middle Eastern Tofu Scramble)

Makes 2 to 4 servings

Shakshuka is traditionally a Middle Eastern breakfast dish made with eggs and tomatoes, kind of like a ragout. Tofu easily replaces the eggs and makes this scramble an herbed, warm, and decadent dish to whip up on a weekend morning. Serve with bread, pitas, or tortillas to round out the meal.

½ cup chopped red onion
½ cup chopped red bell pepper or jarred roasted red bell pepper
½ cup chopped fresh tomatoes
½ cup vegetable stock
1 (14-ounce) package firm or extra-firm tofu, cubed
1 tablespoon tamari
1 tablespoon nutritional yeast
1 teaspoon turmeric
1 teaspoon sweet paprika
¼ teaspoon ground cumin
¼ teaspoon crushed red pepper flakes
½ cup minced fresh dill
½ cup minced fresh Italian flat-leaf parsley
¼ to ½ teaspoon freshly ground black pepper
1 to 2 cups chopped Swiss chard or other leafy green

1. In a large pan over medium-high heat, saute the onion, bell pepper, and tomato in vegetable stock, stirring frequently, until soft, 3 to 5 minutes.

2. Add the tofu, tamari, nutritional yeast, turmeric, paprika, cumin, and red pepper flakes, and cook, stirring frequently, until well-incorporated, 5 minutes.

3. Add the dill, parsley, pepper and chard and cook until greens are wilted, 2 to 3 minutes. Serve hot or store in an airtight container in the refrigerator for up to 3 to 4 days.

Cheesy Smoky Butternut Squash Pasta

Makes 4 to 6 servings

Nothing feels more like comfort food than pasta smothered in a warm, creamy, cheesy sauce and tossed with some sweet, hearty, lightly cooked broccoli. This quickly became a favorite in our home and, thankfully, frozen butternut squash is available so this dish can be enjoyed throughout the seasons.

> 1½ cups chopped butternut squash, raw
> 1 (12-ounce) package dry pasta (e.g., rigatoni, penne, macaroni, and spirals)
> 1½ cups raw broccoli florets
> ¾ cup unsweetened almond, soy, or other plant milk
> ½ cup raw cashews, soaked and drained, or hempseeds
> ½ cup nutritional yeast
> 2 tablespoons freshly squeezed lemon juice with zest
> 1 tablespoon tamari
> ½ to ¾ teaspoon ground chipotle powder

1. Preheat the oven to 375°F.

2. On a baking pan, roast the squash until dark brown and bubbling, 20 minutes.

3. Fill a large pot ¾ full of cold water and bring to a boil over high heat. Once boiling, add pasta and return to a boil. Then, reduce heat and simmer over medium heat until pasta is soft, 20 to 30 minutes. Before draining, add fresh broccoli florets and allow to wilt, 2 to 4 minutes. Drain and return to pot.

4. Meanwhile, puree the squash, almond milk, cashews, nutritional yeast, lemon juice and zest, tamari, and chipotle powder in the blender

until smooth, 10 to 20 seconds. Pour the squash sauce over the pasta and the broccoli, and stir to combine. Serve warm.

Falafel   *Makes 8 to 10 servings (about 56 medium-size falafels)*

This classic Middle Eastern dish is made from mashed beans and spices, deep-fried, and served in pita with hummus, tahini, and Israeli salad. This no-oil version maintains the freshness of the herbs and makes for a much healthified patty to enjoy anytime. This recipe uses dried chickpeas for optimal results, so it requires a bit of advance preparation, with overnight soaking, but the results are worth it.

1 (16-ounce) package dried chickpeas
½ teaspoon baking soda
1 medium-size whole-grain French roll
1 large yellow onion, chopped into quarters
2 bunches fresh cilantro, stems removed
4 to 5 garlic cloves, minced
2 teaspoons baking powder
Pinch of salt, or more to taste (optional)
1 teaspoon crushed red pepper flakes
2 teaspoons ground cumin

1. Soak the chickpeas and baking soda in a large bowl with water double the height of the chickpeas overnight. (See note.)

2. Soak the roll in enough water to soften, 5 minutes. Squeeze water out well and set aside.

3. In a food processor, place the chickpeas mixture, onion, cilantro, garlic, baking powder, salt, red pepper flakes, and cumin, and process until smooth and can be formed into a flat ball with your hands, 1 to 2 minutes.

4. Heat a frying pan until hot, 1 minute. In your hands, take a large tablespoon-sized amount of the batter and flip back and forth to form a flat meatball. Add the flat falafel ball to the pan and cook over medium-high heat until browned on the bottom and firm enough to move, 1 minute. Flip over and cook until browned on the other side, 1 minute. Remove to a dish. Continue process until all the batter is cooked.

5. Serve immediately in a pita with tahini and salad vegetables, if desired or store in an airtight container in the refrigerator for up to 3 to 4 days.

Note: For a shortcut, boil water and pour over the chickpeas to soak for only 2 hours. For an alternative cooking method, place uncooked falafel patties onto a silicon baking sheet or a baking sheet lined with parchment paper, and bake in a preheated oven at 400°F for 10 minutes; flip and bake 5 more minutes.

Green *Ful* *Makes 4 to 6 servings*

A classic ingredient in the Mediterranean, fava beans are also known as "broad beans." Cooked together with potatoes and fresh herbs to make it green, this recipe is delicious and hearty enough to help maintain satiety for hours. Shelling the fava beans requires a bit of extra work, but they taste great fresh. You can also use frozen, if preferred.

2 pounds fresh in-pod fava beans, (about 4 cups shelled)
1½ cups chopped yellow onion
2 small Yukon gold potatoes, peeled and halved
¼ cup vegetable stock
1 cup chopped fresh cilantro
¼ cup chopped fresh dill
2 (8-ounce) cans tomato sauce
3 garlic cloves, minced
1 tablespoon turmeric
1 tablespoon ground cumin
1 tablespoon sweet paprika
1 teaspoon crushed red pepper flakes (optional)

1. Shell fava beans from their pods and place them in a colander to rinse. Slice up 3 or 4 of the pods finely and place them with the beans. Rinse everything well.

2. In a medium pan, saute the onion and potatoes in vegetable stock over medium-high heat until onion is translucent, 5 minutes. Add the fava beans, pods, cilantro, and dill, and cook over medium-high heat until they soften, 2 minutes.

3. Add tomato sauce, garlic, turmeric, cumin, paprika, and red pepper flakes, and bring to a boil. Once boiling, reduce heat and simmer until bubbling, 15 minutes. Serve warm with rice, if desired or store in an airtight container in the refrigerator for up to 4 to 5 days.

Ful Medames (Crushed Fava Beans) *Makes 4 to 6 servings*

This Egyptian dish is traditionally eaten for breakfast with pita bread. It tastes and feels like mashed potatoes, but it is packed with nutrition. Two shortcuts are either to boil water and pour over fava beans to soak for only 2 hours or to use canned fava beans. (If using canned, do not soak or use baking soda.) I love this dish with nutritional yeast flakes sprinkled in for a cheesy flavor and some hot sauce for a kick. Add in as much as you want at the end and stir it up for added deliciousness.

1 (20-ounce) package fava beans
½ teaspoon baking soda
½ teaspoon plus pinch of salt (optional)
3 garlic cloves, minced
1 teaspoon ground cumin
¼ to 1 teaspoon crushed red pepper flakes (optional)
1½ tablespoons freshly squeezed lemon juice, divided with zest
1 large or 2 medium russet potatoes, peeled and roughly chopped
Salt and ground black pepper, to taste
1 to 2 tablespoons chopped fresh parsley for garnish (Note: cilantro or
   other herbs work well here, too)

1. Soak the fava beans with the baking soda in a bowl with water double the height of beans overnight.

2. Rinse and drain the fava bean mixture well. Place in a large pot with fresh water to cover and add the pinch of salt, and bring to a boil over high heat. Once boiling, reduce heat and simmer over low heat until soft enough to mash, 45 to 60 minutes, adding water as needed to keep the beans covered.

3. Meanwhile, in a small bowl, combine garlic, cumin, red pepper flakes, 1 tablespoon lemon juice, and 1/2 teaspoon salt. Set aside.

4. In a medium pot, place the potatoes in enough water to cover and bring to a boil over high heat. Once boiling, reduce heat and cook over medium heat until medium soft, 10 to 15 minutes. Drain and set aside.

5. When the fava beans are cooked, save ½ cup cooking liquid, draining the remaining water. Place the beans back in the pot with the ½ cup reserved cooking liquid. Add the garlic mixture to the beans and bring to a boil over medium-high heat. Reduce heat and simmer until beans are softened, 5 minutes. Turn off the heat. Mash the bean mixture with a potato masher very lightly so the beans are partially mashed.

6. Add the potatoes and remaining lemon juice with zest to the beans. Serve immediately in a bowl with whole-grain pita bread and chopped parsley for garnish, or store in an airtight container in the refrigerator for up to 3 to 4 days.

Mujadara
Makes 2 to 4 servings

Not only is this a popular Arabic dish, but it also happens to be a classic vegetarian recipe since it is the perfect staple. In fact, it is one of the first recipes I mastered when I changed to a plant-based diet several years ago. My mother-in-law Miri makes this simple dish even tastier by adding her incredible garnish that infuses the basic rice and lentils with intensely warm flavor.

MUJADARA
1 medium yellow onion, chopped
¼ cup vegetable stock
2 cups green lentils
2 tablespoons turmeric
1½ tablespoons ground cumin
1 tablespoon freshly ground black pepper
1 teaspoon crushed red pepper flakes
1 garlic clove, minced
1 cup brown basmati rice
Pinch of salt (optional)

GARNISH (optional)
1 large yellow onion, sliced

Peel of 1 orange, thinly sliced
¼ teaspoon ground cinnamon
Pinch of freshly ground black pepper

1. For *Mujadara*, saute the onion in vegetable stock in a medium pot over medium heat until onions are translucent, 5 to 10 minutes. Add lentils and 8 cups water and bring to a boil. Once boiling, reduce heat and simmer until lentils are still firm, for 30 minutes.

2. Add turmeric, cumin, pepper, red pepper flakes, garlic, and rice. Stir to combine and reduce heat to low. Simmer until all water is absorbed, 20 minutes.

3. To prepare garnish, dry-cook onion, orange peel, cinnamon, and pepper in a small pan over medium-high heat. Stir constantly until soft, 4 to 6 minutes.

4. Serve *Mujadara* warm with garnish on top, or store in an airtight container in the refrigerator for up to 4 to 5 days.

Green *Fassulia* (Green Beans) and Potatoes

Makes 2 to 4 servings

Green beans stewed in tomatoes make a great main dish, especially when served with potatoes, softened and savory from soaking up the sauce. This is another perfect synergistic combination of nutrients, with the vitamin C in the tomatoes and lemon juice helping absorb the iron in the beans and the heat promoting carotenoid absorption.

1 cup chopped yellow onion
2 Yukon gold potatoes, peeled and halved
1 cup vegetable stock
1 (16-ounce) package frozen *fassulia* (green beans)
2 garlic cloves
1 tablespoon turmeric
1 teaspoon ground cumin
½ teaspoon freshly ground black pepper
½ teaspoon crushed red pepper flakes
½ teaspoon salt (optional)
1 cup crushed tomatoes
2 tablespoon freshly squeezed lemon juice

1. In a medium pot, saute the onion and potatoes in vegetable stock over medium heat until onion is translucent, 5 to 10 minutes.

2. Add the green beans, garlic, turmeric, cumin, pepper, red pepper flakes, salt, and tomatoes. Bring to a boil. Once boiling, reduce heat and cover. Cover over medium-low heat and simmer until potatoes are soft, 10 minutes.

3. Add lemon juice and cook until sauce is absorbed, 5 more minutes. Serve immediately over rice, if desired, or store in an airtight container in the refrigerator for up to 4 to 5 days.

Hearty Red Lentil Stew   *Makes 6 to 8 servings*

My favorite one-pot wonder, this hearty, earthy, chunky stew explodes with flavor and texture. Enjoy with a piece of Stone-Ground Cornbread and a sprinkle of Parma Shake. This is the perfect meal for entertaining guests or for just feeding a hungry home.

1½ cups chopped yellow onion
1½ cups chopped red bell pepper
1 or 2 garlic cloves, minced
4 cups vegetable stock or water, divided
1½ tablespoons chili powder
1 teaspoon ground cumin
1 teaspoon smoked paprika
½ teaspoon ground chipotle powder
¼ teaspoon crushed red pepper flakes
2 cups red lentils, rinsed
1 (28-ounce) can fire-roasted or plain crushed tomatoes
1 (15-ounce) can chickpeas, drained and rinsed
1 (8-ounce) package tempeh, cubed
2 tablespoons freshly squeezed lemon or lime juice with zest
¼ cup chopped fresh cilantro or Italian flat-leaf parsley for garnish
Pinch of salt and freshly ground black pepper, or more to taste

1. In a large soup pot, saute the onion, bell pepper, and garlic in ½ cup vegetable stock over medium-high heat until onions are translucent, 5 minutes. Add the chili powder, cumin, paprika, chipotle powder, and red pepper flakes, and cook until aromatic, 1 additional minute.

2. Add the lentils, tomatoes, remaining 3½ cups vegetable stock, chickpeas, and tempeh and reduce heat. Cover slightly and bring to a boil. Once boiling, reduce heat and simmer, stirring occasionally, until lentils are soft, 30 minutes.

3. Add the lemon juice and zest, and sprinkle with the cilantro. Add the salt or pepper. Serve warm, or store in an airtight container in the refrigerator for up to 4 to 5 days.

Polenta with Mushroom Ragu   *Makes 4 to 6 servings*

For some reason, I was always intimidated by the idea of making my own polenta. So, I have always used the prepared tubes sold at the store. As it turns out, it is incredibly easy to make, and this version is great as a crust. My favorite addition? Serving it up with mushrooms as a ragu. Together, mushrooms and corn make a dynamic duo, and this dish is pizza-esque.

    3 cups vegetable stock, divided
    1 tablespoon turmeric
    1 teaspoon ground cumin
    Pinch of salt (optional)
    1 cup yellow cornmeal
    1 medium yellow onion, chopped
    3 garlic cloves, minced
    1 (8-ounce) package baby bella or other brown mushrooms, chopped
    1 (8-ounce) package white button mushrooms, chopped
    1 bay leaf
    1 teaspoon dried thyme
    1 teaspoon dried oregano
    ½ cup finely chopped fresh Italian flat-leaf parsley
    1 tablespoon balsamic vinegar
    2 to 4 tablespoons Parma Shake (see page 182 for recipe.)

1. In a medium saucepan over medium-high heat, bring 2 cups vegetable stock, turmeric, cumin, and salt to a boil. Once boiling, add the cornmeal in a steady stream, stirring constantly. Reduce heat and simmer, stirring frequently, until cornmeal thickens, 3 to 5 minutes.

Remove from heat and pour into a 9-inch pie dish, evenly distributing. Cover with plastic wrap and refrigerate until it hardens, 20 minutes.

2. Meanwhile, preheat oven to 350°F.

3. In a medium saucepan, saute the onion and garlic in 1 cup vegetable stock over medium-high heat until onion is translucent, 5 minutes. Add the mushrooms, bay leaf, thyme, and oregano, and cook until all liquid is absorbed, 10 minutes. Turn off heat, remove the bay leaf, and add the parsley and balsamic vinegar.

4. Take the polenta out of the refrigerator and sprinkle on Parma Shake. Bake until lightly browned, 10 minutes. Remove from the oven and spoon the mushroom ragu evenly atop the polenta. Slice into pie slices and serve warm, or store in an airtight container in the refrigerator for up to 4 to 5 days.

Moussaka   *Makes 6 to 8 servings*

Moussaka is a traditional layered casserole baked dish, made with eggplant and usually a meat filling. Here, red lentils and mushrooms provide the ground round texture to make this Vegiterranean. Moussaka is one of the most popular Greek dishes, and we can see why when we enjoy this intricate combination that is both filling and, surprisingly, not heavy.

1 large eggplant, sliced into ½-inch-thick rounds

FILLING
1 cup green lentils, rinsed
1 yellow onion, chopped
¼ cup vegetable stock
2 cups chopped mushrooms
¼ cup chopped fresh cilantro, stems removed
1 garlic clove, minced
1 teaspoon freshly ground black pepper
1 teaspoon ground cumin
1 teaspoon turmeric
½ teaspoon crushed red pepper flakes
½ teaspoon salt (optional)
1½ teaspoons egg replacer

SAUCE
1 cup crushed tomatoes
1 teaspoon turmeric
1 teaspoon ground cumin
1 teaspoon crushed red pepper flakes

GARNISH
½ cup finely chopped fresh basil

1. Preheat the oven to 400°F.

2. On a baking sheet lined with a silicone liner or parchment paper, place eggplant slices in a single layer. Bake until lightly browned, 20 minutes. Flip them and bake until lightly browned, 10 more minutes. Remove from the oven but leave the heat on.

3. Meanwhile, place the lentils and 4 cups of water in a medium pot. Cover and bring to a boil over medium-high heat. Once boiling, reduce heat and simmer over medium-low heat until lentils are tender, 20 to 30 minutes. When lentils are soft, remove from heat, strain, and set aside.

4. For the filling, in a separate medium pan, saute the onion in vegetable stock over medium-high heat until onion is translucent, 5 minutes. Add the mushrooms, cilantro, garlic, pepper, cumin, turmeric, red pepper flakes, and salt, and cook until the mushrooms are soft, 5 minutes. Add the lentils and cook over medium heat until most of the liquid is absorbed, 5 minutes. Sprinkle in the egg replacer and stir to combine. Cook until mixture thickens. Turn off heat.

5. For the sauce, combine tomatoes, turmeric, cumin, and red pepper flakes in a small dish.

6. In a 9 x 13-inch baking dish, layer half the eggplant slices on the bottom. Add the filling on top of the eggplant and cover with the remaining eggplant slices. Top with the sauce and the basil. Cover the dish with aluminum foil and bake until all liquid is absorbed, 10 minutes. Remove the aluminum foil and bake until lightly browned, 10 more minutes. Serve hot, or store in an airtight container in the refrigerator for up to 4 to 5 days.

Dolci (Sweets)

Fruit is a perfect dessert when a sweet tooth calls, and it is what was traditionally enjoyed in the Mediterranean. Light, seasonal, and nutrient-dense, there is nothing sweet that compares to fruit. Blended frozen fruit is excellent in the summer as a cold treat and served fresh or cooked—such as grilled, stewed, or poached fruits, pies, compotes, and crumbles—in the colder months. For some occasions, when we are craving something a bit more elaborate, here are some wholesome—yet still decadent—options!

Chocolate Hazelnut Chia Pudding   *Makes 4 servings*

Ch-ch-ch … chia with ch-ch-ch … chocolate and combined with hazelnut is a decadent match made in heaven, especially when it is healthy, too—the chia seeds add protein and omega-3s! This creamy dark chocolate pudding has a nutty essence and is fun to eat with the tapioca-like texture from the chia seeds.

> 2 cups plain unsweetened almond, soy, or other plant milk
> 3 tablespoons pure cacao (cocoa) powder
> 2 tablespoons hazelnuts
> 6 to 8 medium sized dates
> 1 teaspoon alcohol-free vanilla extract
> 6 tablespoons chia seeds

1. Puree the plant milk, cacao powder, hazelnuts, dates, and vanilla in a blender until smooth, 20 to 30 seconds. Add the chia seeds and slowly blend on low just until combined, 5 to 10 seconds. Allow mixture to sit in blender for 5 minutes. Then, slowly blend once again to combine.

2. Pour the pudding into individual cups and refrigerate to allow chia to swell, at least 1 hour, or store in an airtight container in the refrigerator for up to 2 to 3 days.

Italian Wedding Cookies

Makes 12 cookies

RECIPE BY ROBIN ROBERTSON

Also known variously as Mexican Wedding Cookies and Russian Tea Cookies, these tasty bites are usually made with lots of butter. With its emphasis on simple, whole ingredients, this version gives you all the flavor without all the added fat.

1 cup chopped walnuts
½ cup plus 2 tablespoons coconut flour, divided
¼ cup golden raisins, soaked and drained
Pinch of salt
¼ cup pure maple syrup
2 tablespoons almond milk, or more, as needed

1. Preheat the oven to 300°F. Line a baking sheet with parchment paper and set aside.

2. Place the walnuts in a food processor and pulse until finely ground, 10 to 20 seconds. Add ½ cup coconut flour, raisins, and salt. Pulse to combine, 10 to 20 seconds. Add the maple syrup and the almond milk, and pulse until the dough starts to hold together, 10 to 20 seconds. (Add an additional 1 tablespoon almond milk, if needed, to help the dough come together.)

3. Divide the dough into four equal portions, then divide each portion into three equal pieces to make 12 portions. Roll each portion into a ball and flatten slightly.

4. Arrange the cookies on the prepared baking sheet. Bake until the cookies look dry and lightly browned, 12 minutes. Cool on a cooling rack completely before handling.

5. When the cookies are cool, place the remaining 2 tablespoons of coconut flour in a small bowl. Add the cookies to the bowl, 1 or 2 at a time, and roll them around to coat. Repeat with the remaining cookies.

Summer Fruit Tart

Makes 8 servings

RECIPE BY ROBIN ROBERTSON

This easy and versatile no-bake tart features a date-and-nut crust with a layer of mango puree and topped with a variety of fresh fruits.

CRUST
1 cup chopped walnuts
½ cup cashews
⅛ teaspoon salt
½ cup pitted dates

TOPPINGS
1 ripe fresh mango, peeled and diced
2 cups fresh strawberries, hulled and sliced
1 medium ripe kiwifruit, peeled and thinly sliced
½ cup fresh blueberries
Small fresh mint leaves for garnish (optional)

1. For the crust, combine the walnuts, cashews, and salt in a food processor and pulse until finely ground, 10 to 20 seconds. Add the dates and pulse until well incorporated and the mixture begins to stick together, 10 to 20 seconds.

2. Transfer to a 9-inch tart pan with a removable bottom. Press firmly and evenly onto the bottom of the pan. Place the pan in the refrigerator or freezer while you prepare the mango puree.

3. For the toppings, place the mango in a food processor and puree until smooth, 5 to 10 seconds. Spread the mango puree over the crust, leaving a ½-inch border along the perimeter of the crust.

4. Arrange the strawberries, kiwifruit, and blueberries decoratively on top of the mango puree. Chill in the refrigerator until ready to serve. To serve, garnish with mint leaves and cut the tart into wedges.

Ganache Parfait with Poached Berries

Makes 6 to 8 servings

RECIPE BY CHAD SARNO

This rich and decadent dessert is perfect for the chocoholic at your dinner party. Serve this almond ganache as a dip for fresh fruits, as a frosting for cakes, piped into cannoli, served with crèpes, spread on toast, or as a layer in a show-stopping dessert.

Berries and port could not pair better. This raw dessert compote kicks your desserts over the top. If you are looking to swap out the alcohol, fresh pomegranate is a great substitution. Use on your favorite non-dairy gelato or ice cream, or serve as a layer in parfaits.

ALMOND GANACHE
¾ cup raw almond butter
1 cup date paste
¼ cup maple syrup
½ tablespoon tamari
2 teaspoons vanilla extract
1 cup unsweetened cocoa powder
½ cup coconut water, or more as needed

POACHED BERRIES
4 cups fresh berries, (if using raspberries, halve, and strawberries, quarter)
1¼ cups port
Juice of ½ lime
¼ cup maple syrup
1 full vanilla bean, scraped (or 1 teaspoon vanilla extract)
½ teaspoon sea salt

PARFAITS
½ cup crushed pecans, toasted

1. To make the ganache, place the almond butter, date paste, maple syrup, tamari, vanilla, cocoa powder, and coconut water in food processor and blend well until smooth, 5 to 10 seconds. (It may be difficult to blend

at first so add more coconut water as needed to create a smooth frosting-like consistency.) Set aside.

2. For the poached berries, in medium mixing bowl, toss the berries, port, lime juice, maple syrup, vanilla, and salt well and very gently; you want the berries to remain intact.

3. Let stand, tossing gently occasionally, to marry all the flavors, at least 1 hour.

4. Make the parfaits in 6 to 8 small parfait glasses, starting with a layer of poached berries, followed by ganache; repeat layering. Top with a sprinkle of pecans.

Note: To make date paste, puree 1 cup pitted dates with ¼ cup water in a blender to make a thick paste.

Grilled Nectarines with Amaretto Gelato

Makes 4 to 5 servings
(Makes 2½ cups gelato)

RECIPE BY CHAD SARNO

Grilling stone fruits such as peaches, nectarines, and apricots allows the sugars to caramelize and natural sweetness to be highlighted in this light and refreshing dessert. With the sweet acidity of the balsamic glaze, these gems are paired for success with this rich and decadent amaretto gelato. Grilled fruits can be used for sweet or savory recipes.

Looking for that sweet, rich, and decadent gelato without the moo? Look no further; this coconut-and-cashew-based dessert is great as a gelato or highlighted simply as a sweet finishing cream for fresh or grilled fruits.

AMARETTO GELATO
1¼ cups raw cashews
1 cup canned coconut milk
¼ cup amaretto
½ teaspoon almond extract
⅓ cup maple syrup
Pinch of sea salt

GRILLED NECTARINES
3 tablespoons good-quality white balsamic vinegar

3 tablespoons maple syrup
⅛ teaspoon freshly ground nutmeg
¼ teaspoon freshly ground black pepper
¼ teaspoon sea salt
4 slightly ripe, but not soft nectarines or peaches, halved and pitted

1. For the gelato, soak the cashews in enough water to cover until softened, 2 hours.

2. In a blender, blend the cashews, coconut milk, amaretto, almond extract, maple syrup, and salt, folding as necessary with a rubber spatula to ensure a smooth consistency, 10 to 20 seconds.

3. Using an ice cream maker, follow the manufacturer's instructions and process the mixture. Alternatively, this is a delicious cream served with the grilled nectarines or fruit of your choice.

4. Prepare a hot grill on high, and once hot, reduce to medium heat.

5. For the grilled nectarines, whisk together the vinegar, maple syrup, nutmeg, pepper, and salt in a small bowl. Using a pastry brush, brush the vinegar mixture over the flesh side of the nectarines.

6. Place the nectarines cut-side down on the grill and grill, occasionally drizzling a little bit of the glaze over the top of the nectarines, until lightly browned, 3 to 4 minutes. (If using a grill pan, make sure your fan is on, as this may be smoky.)

7. Remove the nectarines from the grill, and spoon Amaretto Gelato into the hollows of the nectarines. Serve immediately.

Chocolate Crispy Fruit Squares *Makes 9 to 12 squares*

A happy compromise between an energy bar and a decadent dessert, these crispy, chewy, sweet squares are delightful and can be enjoyed however you prefer. Kid friendly, dietitian-approved, these treats are perfect for on-the-go.

1 cup dates
1 cup raisins
½ cup chopped walnuts
2 tablespoons sesame seeds
¼ cup dairy-free dark chocolate chips (grain-sweetened, if possible)
1 cup puffed rice cereal

1. In a food processor, puree the dates and the raisins until smooth, 20 to 30 seconds. Add the walnuts and the sesame seeds, and process until combined, 10 to 20 seconds. Pulse in the chocolate chips and then the cereal. In between additions, use a spatula or a wooden spoon to break up the ball and to incorporate the other ingredients.

2. Transfer the mixture to a silicon or glass 8 x 8-inch square dish, and press firmly and evenly into the dish. Cover and refrigerate until hardened, at least 1 hour. Cut into bars and serve immediately or store in an airtight container in the refrigerator for up 4 to 5 days.

Note: Alternatively, the mixture can be rolled into spheres, and then refrigerated and served.

Resources

WEBSITES

Nutrition:

Brenda Davis: brendadavisrd.com

Dietary Reference Intakes: fnic.nal.usda.gov/dietary-guidance/dietary-reference-intakes

Recommended Dietary Allowance and Adequate Intake Values or Vitamins, Elements, Total Water and Macronutrients tables, and Tolerable Upper Intake Level Values for Vitamins and Elements table from: http://www.iom.edu/Activities/Nutrition/SummaryDRIs/DRI-Tables.aspx

Linus Pauling Institute's Micronutrient Information Center: lpi.oregonstate.edu/infocenter/

Ginny Messina: theveganrd.com

Nutrition Facts: nutritionfacts.org

Plant-Based Dietitian: plantbaseddietitian.com

Plant-Based Research: plantbasedresearch.org

Physicians Committee for Responsible Medicine: pcrm.org

USDA National Nutrient Database for Standard Reference: ndb.nal.usda.gov

Vegan Health: veganhealth.org

Vegetarian Nutrition Dietetic Practice Group of the Academy of Nutrition and Dietetics: vegetariannutrition.net/faq

Veganism:

Carnism Awareness and Action Network (CAAN): carnism.org

Farm Sanctuary: farmsanctuary.org

HappyCow: happycow.net

Mercy for Animals: mercyforanimals.org

VegNews: vegnews.com

BOOKS

21-Day Weight Loss Kickstart, Neal Barnard, Grand Central Life & Style, 2013

Becoming Raw, Brenda Davis and Vesanto Melina, Book Publishing Company, 2010

Becoming Vegan: Express Edition and *Becoming Vegan: Comprehensive Edition,* Brenda Davis and Vesanto Melina, Book Publishing Company, 2013 and 2014, respectively

Diet for a New America, 25th Anniversary Edition, John Robbins, HJ Kramer/New World Library, 2012

Disease-Proof Your Child, Joel Fuhrman, St. Martin's Griffin, 2006

Dr. Neal Barnard's Program for Reversing Diabetes, Neal Barnard, Rodale Books, 2008

Food Choice and Sustainability, Richard Oppenlander, Langdon Street Press, 2013

Main Street Vegan, Victoria Moran, Tarcher, 2012

Salt, Sugar, Fat, Michael Moss, Random House, 2013

The Blue Zones, Second Edition: 9 Lessons for Living Longer From the People Who've Lived the Longest Dan Buettner, National Geographic, 2012

The China Study, T. Colin Campbell and Thomas M. Campbell II, BenBella Books, 2006

The Complete Idiot's Guide to Plant-Based Nutrition, Julieanna Hever, Alpha Penguin, 2011

The End of Overeating, David A. Kessler, Rodale, 2009

The Food Revolution, John Robbins, Conari Press, 2010

The Pleasure Trap, Douglas J. Lisle and Alan Goldhamer, Book Publishing Company, 2006

Vegan for Life, Jack Norris and Virginia Messina, Da Capo Lifelong Books, 2011

Whole: Rethinking the Science of Nutrition, T. Colin Campbell, BenBella Books, 2013

Why Calories Count, Marion Nestle and Malden Nesheim, University of California Press, 2012

Why We Love Dogs, Eat Pigs, and Wear Cows, Melanie Joy, Conari Press, 2010

COOKBOOKS

1,000 Vegan Recipes, Robin Robertson, Houghton Mifflin Harcourt, 2009

Artisan Vegan Cheese, Miyoko Schinner, Book Publishing Company, 2012

One-Dish Vegan, Robin Robertson, Harvard Common Press, 2013

Let Them Eat Vegan, Dreena Burton, Da Capo Press, 2012

Plant-Powered Families, Dreena Burton, Benbella, 2015

The Complete Idiot's Guide to Gluten-Free Vegan Cooking, Julieanna Hever and Beverly Lynn Bennett, Alpha Penguin, 2011

Nutrients Charts and Tables

Detailed and updated Institute of Medicine Dietary Reference Intakes (recommended dietary allowances, RDAs; estimated average requirement, EARs; adequate intake, AIs, all of which are followed by an asterisk (*); and tolerable upper intake, UI) for all of the vitamins, minerals, and macronutrients can be found online.[1] Below are the RDAs for the nutrients emphasized throughout this book.

Protein RDA:

Age	RDA Protein (g/kg/d)
Ages 0 to 1 year	1.5
Ages 1 to 3 years	1.1
Ages 4 to 13 years	0.95
Ages 14 to 18 years	0.85
Ages 19 and above	0.8
Pregnant (using pre-pregnancy weight)	1.1
Lactating	1.1

FAT-SOLUBLE VITAMINS

Vitamin A Requirements

Age	RDA/AI* (mcg RAE per day)**	Upper Level Intake (mcg RAE per day)
0 to 6 months	400	600
7 to 12 months	500	600
1 to 3 years	300	600
4 to 8 years	400	900
9 to 13 years	600	1,700
Males:		
14 to 18 years	900	2,800
≥19 years	900	3,000

Vitamin A Requirements

Age	RDA/AI* (mcg RAE per day)**	Upper Level Intake (mcg RAE per day)
Females:		
14 to 18 years	700	2,800
≥19 years	700	3,000
Pregnancy:		
≤18 years	750	2,800
≥19 years	770	3,000
Lactation:		
≤18 years	1,200	2,800
≥19 years	1,300	3,000

**RAE means "retinol activity equivalents" where 1 RAE = 1 microgram retinol

Vitamin D Requirements

Age	RDA/AI* (IU per day)	Upper Level Intake (IU per day)
0 to 6 months	400	1,000
7 to 12 months	400	1,500
1 to 3 years	600	2,500
4 to 8 years	600	3,000
9 to 13 years	600	4,000
14 to 18 years	600	4,000
19 to 30 years	600	4,000
31 to 50 years	600	4,000
51 to 70 years	600	4,000
>70 years	800	4,000
Pregnant	600	4,000
Lactating	600	4,000

Vitamin E Requirements

Age	RDA/AI* (milligrams per day)
0 to 6 months	4*
7 to 12 months	5*
1 to 3 years	6
4 to 8 years	7
9 to 13 years	11
14 and older	15
Pregnancy	15
Lactation	19

Vitamin K Requirements

Age	RDA/AI* (micrograms per day)
0 to 6 months	2.0*
7 to 12 months	2.5*
1 to 3 years	30*
4 to 8 years	55*
Males:	
9 to 13 years	60*
14 to 18 years	75*
19 and older	120*
Females:	
9 to 13 years	60*
14 to 18 years	75*
19 and older	90*
Pregnancy and Lactation	
≤ 18 years	75*
19 and older	90*

WATER-SOLUBLE VITAMINS

Thiamin (Vitamin B1) Requirements:

Age	RDA/AI* (milligrams per day)
0 to 6 months	0.2*
7 to 12 months	0.3*
1 to 3 years	0.5
4 to 8 years	0.6
Males:	
9 to 13 years	0.9
14 and older	1.2
Females:	
9 to 13 years	0.9
14 to 18 years	1.0
19 and older	1.1
Pregnancy and Lactation	1.4

Riboflavin (Vitamin B2) Requirements:

Age	RDA/AI* (milligrams per day)
0 to 6 months	0.3*
7 to 12 months	0.4*
1 to 3 years	0.5
4 to 8 years	0.6
Males:	
9 to 13 years	0.9
14 and older	1.3
Females:	
9 to 13 years	0.9
14 to 18 years	1.0
19 and older	1.1
Pregnancy	1.4
Lactation	1.6

Niacin (Vitamin B3) Requirements:

Age	RDA/AI* (milligrams per day)
0 to 6 months	2*
7 to 12 months	4*
1 to 3 years	6
4 to 8 years	8
Males:	
9 to 13 years	12
14 and older	16
Females:	
9 to 13 years	12
14 and older	14
Pregnancy	18
Lactation	17

Pyridoxine (Vitamin B6) Requirements:

Age	RDA/AI* (milligrams per day)
0 to 6 months	0.1*
7 to 12 months	0.3*
1 to 3 years	0.5
4 to 8 years	0.6
Males:	
9 to 13 years	1.0
14 to 50	1.3
50 and older	1.7
Females:	
9 to 13 years	1.0
14 to 18 years	1.2
19 to 50 years	1.3
50 and older	1.5
Pregnancy	1.9
Lactation	2.0

Pantothenic acid (Vitamin B5) Requirements:

Age	RDA/AI* (milligrams per day)
0 to 6 months	1.7*
7 to 12 months	1.8*
1 to 3 years	2*
4 to 8 years	3*
9 to 13 years	4*
14 and older	5*
Pregnancy	6*
Lactation	7*

Biotin (Vitamin B7) Requirements:

Age	RDA/AI* (milligrams per day)
0 to 6 months	5*
7 to 12 months	6*
1 to 3 years	8*
4 to 8 years	12*
9 to 13 years	20*
14 to 18 years	25*
19 and older	30*
Pregnancy	30*
Lactation	35*

Folate (Vitamin B9) Requirements:

Age	RDA/AI* (micrograms per day)
0 to 6 months	65*
7 to 12 months	80*
1 to 3 years	150
4 to 8 years	200
9 to 13 years	300
14 and older	400
Pregnancy	600
Lactation	500

Choline Requirements:

Age	RDA/AI* (milligrams per day)
0 to 6 months	125*
7 to 12 months	150*
1 to 3 years	200*
4 to 8 years	250*
Males:	
9 to 13 years	375*
14 and older	550*
Females:	
9 to 13 years	375*
14 to 18 years	400*
19 and older	425*
Pregnancy	450*
Lactation	550*

Vitamin B12 Requirements:

Age	RDA/AI* (micrograms per day)
0 to 6 months	0.4
6 to 12 months	0.5
1 to 3 years	0.9
4 to 8 years	1.2
9 to 13 years	1.8
14 and older	2.4
Pregnant	2.6
Lactation	2.8

Vitamin C Requirements:

Age	RDA/AI* (milligrams per day)
0 to 6 months	40*
7 to 12 months	50*
1 to 3 years	15
4 to 8 years	25
Males:	
9 to 13 years	45
14 to 18 years	75
19 and older	90
Females:	
9 to 13 years	45
14 to 18 years	65
19 and older	75
Pregnancy	
≤ 18 years	80
19 and older	85
Lactation	
≤ 18 years	115
19 and older	120

MINERALS

Calcium Requirements:

Age	RDA/AI* (milligrams per day)
0 to 6 months	210*
7 to 12 months	270*
1 to 3 years	500*
4 to 8 years	800*
9 to 18 years	1,300*
19 to 50 years	1,000*
50 and older	1,200*
Pregnancy and Lactation	
≤ 18 years	1,300*
19 and older	1,000*

Iodine Requirements:

Age	RDA/AI* (micrograms per day)
0 to 6 months	110*
7 to 12 months	130*
1 to 3 years	90
4 to 8 years	90
9 to 13 years	120
14 and older	150
Pregnancy	220
Lactation	290

Iron Requirements:

Age	RDA/AI* (milligrams per day)
0 to 6 months	0.27*
7 to 12 months	11
1 to 3 years	7
4 to 8 years	10
Males:	
9 to 13 years	8
14 to 18 years	11
19 and older	8
Females:	
9 to 13 years	8
14 to 18 years	15
19 to 50 years	18
50 and older	8
Pregnancy	27
Lactation:	
≤ 18 years	10
19 and older	9

Magnesium Requirements:

Age	RDA/AI* (milligrams per day)
0 to 6 months	30*
7 to 12 months	75*
1 to 3 years	80
4 to 8 years	130
Males:	
9 to 13 years	240
14 to 18 years	410
19 to 30 years	400
31 and older	420
Females:	
9 to 13 years	240
14 to 18 years	360
19 to 30 years	310
31 and older	320
Pregnancy:	
≤ 18 years	400
19 to 30 years	350
31 to 50 years	360
Lactation:	
≤ 18 years	360
19 to 30 years	310
31 to 50 years	320

Potassium Requirements:

Age	RDA/AI* (grams per day)
0 to 6 months	0.4*
7 to 12 months	0.7*
1 to 3 years	3.0*
4 to 8 years	3.8*
9 to 13 years	4.5*
14 and older	4.7*
Pregnancy	4.7*
Lactation	5.1*

Selenium Requirements:

Age	RDA/AI* (micrograms per day)
0 to 6 months	15*
7 to 12 months	20*
1 to 3 years	20
4 to 8 years	30
9 to 13 years	40
14 and older	55
Pregnancy	60
Lactation	70

Sodium Requirements:

Age	RDA/AI* (grams per day)
0 to 6 months	0.12*
7 to 12 months	0.37*
1 to 3 years	1.0*
4 to 8 years	1.2*
9 to 50 years	1.5*
50 to 70 years	1.3*
70 and older	1.2*
Pregnancy and Lactation	1.5*

Zinc Requirements:

Age	RDA/AI* (milligrams per day)
0 to 6 months	2*
7 to 12 months	3
1 to 3 years	3
4 to 8 years	5
Males:	
9 to 13 years	8
14 and older	11
Females:	
9 to 13 years	8
14 to 18 years	9
19 and older	8
Pregnancy:	
≤ 18 years	12
19 and older	11
Lactation:	
≤ 18 years	13
19 and older	12

METRIC CONVERSIONS

- The recipes in this book have not been tested with metric measurements, so some variations might occur.
- Remember that the weight of dry ingredients varies according to the volume or density factor: 1 cup of flour weighs far less than 1 cup of sugar, and 1 tablespoon doesn't necessarily hold 3 teaspoons.

General Formulas for Metric Conversion

Ounces to grams	$\Rightarrow$ ounces × 28.35 = grams
Grams to ounces	$\Rightarrow$ grams × 0.035 = ounces
Pounds to grams	$\Rightarrow$ pounds × 453.5 = grams
Pounds to kilograms	$\Rightarrow$ pounds × 0.45 = kilograms
Cups to liters	$\Rightarrow$ cups × 0.24 = liters
Fahrenheit to Celsius	$\Rightarrow$ (°F − 32) × 5 ÷ 9 = °C
Celsius to Fahrenheit	$\Rightarrow$ (°C × 9) ÷ 5 + 32 = °F

Linear Measurements

½ inch = 1½ cm
1 inch = 2½ cm
6 inches = 15 cm
8 inches = 20 cm
10 inches = 25 cm
12 inches = 30 cm
20 inches = 50 cm

Volume (Dry) Measurements

¼ teaspoon = 1 milliliter
½ teaspoon = 2 milliliters
¾ teaspoon = 4 milliliters
1 teaspoon = 5 milliliters
1 tablespoon = 15 milliliters
¼ cup = 59 milliliters
⅓ cup = 79 milliliters
½ cup = 118 milliliters
⅔ cup = 158 milliliters
¾ cup = 177 milliliters
1 cup = 225 milliliters
4 cups or 1 quart = 1 liter
½ gallon = 2 liters
1 gallon = 4 liters

Volume (Liquid) Measurements

1 teaspoon = ⅙ fluid ounce = 5 milliliters
1 tablespoon = ½ fluid ounce = 15 milliliters
2 tablespoons = 1 fluid ounce = 30 milliliters
¼ cup = 2 fluid ounces = 60 milliliters
⅓ cup = 2⅔ fluid ounces = 79 milliliters
½ cup = 4 fluid ounces = 118 milliliters
1 cup or ½ pint = 8 fluid ounces = 250 milliliters
2 cups or 1 pint = 16 fluid ounces = 500 milliliters
4 cups or 1 quart = 32 fluid ounces = 1,000 milliliters
1 gallon = 4 liters

Oven Temperature Equivalents, Fahrenheit (F) and Celsius (C)

100°F = 38°C
200°F = 95°C
250°F = 120°C
300°F = 150°C
350°F = 180°C
400°F = 205°C
450°F = 230°C

Weight (Mass) Measurements

1 ounce = 30 grams
2 ounces = 55 grams
3 ounces = 85 grams
4 ounces = ¼ pound = 125 grams
8 ounces = ½ pound = 240 grams
12 ounces = ¾ pound = 375 grams
16 ounces = 1 pound = 454 grams

Acknowledgments ... Amore

Dedicated to my Ema Miri, the woman who inspires me to be the best person I can be, and her son—my love—Aviv, who has always supported me steadfastly on my journey ... and, of course, our *piccoli* Vegiterraneans, *Bella* Maya and *Affascinante* Benny ... for filling my heart with love and for always being willing to speak with an Italian (or any other) accent with me.

It quite literally takes a *villaggio* to put together a book, and I am filled with gratitude to my powerful circle of support. Mom, Dad, Nay, Donna, and Abba, thank you for being my biggest cheerleaders and for lending me your ears to bounce off ideas and thoughts. Dennis Mike, your fantastic wit and humor-infused support are priceless.

Renee Sedliar, thank you for your continuous support and for taking on this passion project. Zach Schisgal, my dream-come-true literary agent, who has always had the vision and has held my hand throughout every stage, I am eternally grateful for you. To Diane Perez, my sharp-as-a-tack, inspiring, and astonishing manager, thank you for sharing my hunger to change the world; and thank you, Ryan LeVine, for keeping us safeguarded as we do so. Thank you, Shelly James, for keeping me in alignment, and teaching me about split infinitives, gerunds, antecedents, and then some. Cheers to Marco Pavia for adding such *incanto* to the edits.

One of the greatest honors ever is to have Dr. Neal Barnard contribute the foreword to this book. Dr. Barnard is truly a modern-day hero, by any standard, a man who has singlehandedly improved the fate of humans and animals alike, proving that courage and fortitude mixed with quite a bit of intellect and humor can quite literally save the world.

Thank you to my Soul Mom, Brenda Davis, my mentor, who always generously shares her deep wisdom and intelligence from a place of love and compassion. I am privileged and deeply grateful for your guidance, acumen, and openness. The world is more gorgeous because of you, Brenda.

Dr. Melanie Joy, you are not only a hero of mine, you are one of my closest friends and confidantes. The brilliance you radiate enlightens anyone who is fortunate enough to cross your path. Your ingenious work is inspiring a new paradigm, and I am appreciative to be a witness.

Thank you, Dr. Richard Oppenlander, for setting forth to enumerate the innumerable, for illustrating the depth of imminence facing society, and for being brave and bold about teaching us. Your words in this book are priceless.

To the lifesaver, Gene Baur, for finding a way to protect the innocents, for shedding a hopeful light on the dark, and for inspiring so many to do the same.

Gratitude to Dr. T. Colin Campbell, the Father of Modern Nutrition, for pioneering a new generation of nutritional thought, for allowing me to help share your work, and for defining the whole food, plant-based diet.

I am appreciative for the work of Dr. Marion Nestle, a true scientist with excellent and smart intention. Thank you for sharing your knowledge and for uncovering the hidden truths behind our plates.

Dr. Michael Greger—the walking encyclopedia and role model—enlightens me along with hundreds of thousands of people to seek the truth and to mind the heart, in the meanwhile. Thank you, Dr. Greger, for answering my stressful calls for confirmation and for keeping me—and the world—attuned to the latest in science in the most entertaining way.

Much gratitude to the wise and prolific Ginny Messina, the vegan nutrition expert who has set the standard for being accountable to facts, science, and the pursuit of a compassionate—yet accurate—truth.

Jack Norris, thank you for having answers, charts, and tables to help us all see that we can not only survive—but thrive—without harming animals.

Chad Sarno, thank you for sharing your culinary excellence with your delicious, awe-inspiring recipes. Huge gratitude to Robin Robertson, a woman whose cuisine creativeness is infinite and marvelous, for her recipe contribution. Sherri Nestorowich, thank you for creating pyramids, plates, and other illustrations with such insight and talent.

To Lisa Bloom, love and gratitude for personifying valor, grace, and, sparkle, inspiring me to see no limits. And to my dear friend and role model, Dreena Burton, thank you for teaching and encouraging me about the culinary beauty of foods and for being such a delicious light in this world. And thank you, Catherine Linard, for helping me find my "capital T-truth."

About the Author

Julieanna Hever, M.S., R.D., C.P.T. is a Registered Dietitian who specializes in weight management, disease prevention and management, and sports nutrition. Julieanna is the host of the wellness talk show series *What Would Julieanna Do?* on Veria Living Network, author of the best-selling book, *The Complete Idiot's Guide to Plant-Based Nutrition*, and the nutrition columnist for *VegNews* Magazine. She is the co-author of the cookbook, *The Complete Idiot's Guide to Gluten-Free Vegan Cooking* and a recipe contributor to both *New York Times* bestselling *Forks Over Knives* books. Julieanna counsels a variety of clients throughout the world from her Los Angeles, California-based private practice including elite athletes, adults, and children with various nutritional and/or medical concerns. She is published in prominent journals, magazines, blogs, and newsletters. Julieanna has served as a Special Consultant for the bestselling documentary, *Forks Over Knives* and as the Executive Director of *EarthSave, International*.

Julieanna received her Bachelors degree from UCLA and Masters of Science in Nutrition at California State University, Northridge, where she also completed her Dietetic Internship. She has taught as part of Dr. T. Colin Campbell's eCornell Plant-Based Nutrition Certification Program, worked as a clinical dietitian at Century City Doctors Hospital, and has consulted for numerous businesses.

To learn more, visit Julieanna at her website: PlantBasedDietitian.com

ABOUT THE RECIPE CONTRIBUTORS

Chad Sarno has brought his unique culinary style to a vast array of projects throughout his career before joining Rouxbe Online Culinary School as VP of Plant-Based Education. Spanning from the launch of a boutique plant-based restaurant brand throughout Europe in Istanbul, London and Munich, to the development of innovative health and wellness initiatives as culinary media spokesperson for Whole Foods Market's global healthy eating program,

Chad's mission of health inspired plant-based eating has reached all corners of the globe.

Chad has been contributing chef to numerous recipe books as well as featured in many national publications. He has been a guest on dozens of morning shows and food-focused programs on television and radio internationally over the years. Through the intersection of clean food and culinary education, Chad continues to share his passion for helping others achieve their health goals, starting in the kitchen.

In 2012, Chad has teamed up with best selling author, Kris Carr to write the New York Times Best Seller, *Crazy Sexy Kitchen*.

For more information on Chad's work visit: chadsarno.com and for online plant-based courses visit rouxbe.com/plant-based.

Robin Robertson has written more than twenty cookbooks, including the best-sellers *Vegan Planet, Quick-Fix Vegan, 1,000 Vegan Recipes, Fresh from the Vegan Slow Cooker,* and *One-Dish Vegan.* A longtime vegan and former restaurant chef, she has written for VegNews Magazine, Vegetarian Times, Cooking Light, and other magazines. Robin's Web site is robinrobertson.com.

Notes

CHAPTER 1

1. Serra-Majem, Lluis, Blanca Roman, and Ramon Estruch. "Scientific evidence of interventions using the Mediterranean diet: a systematic review." *Nutrition Reviews* 64, no. 2 (2006): S27-S47.

2. Allbaugh, Leland. *Crete*. Princeton: Princeton University Press, 1953.

3. Allbaugh, Leland G. *Crete: a case study of an underdeveloped area*. New Jersey: Princeton University Press, 1953.

4. Ibid.

5. Andrade, Jason, Aneez Mohamed, Jiri Frohlich, and Andrew Ignaszewski. "Ancel Keys and the lipid hypothesis: From early breakthroughs to current management of dyslipidemia." *BC Medical Journal* 51, no. 2 (2009): 66-72.

6. Keys, Ancel, Henry Longstreet Taylor, Henry Blackburn, Jodef Brozek, Joseph T. Anderson, and Ernst Simonson. "Coronary Heart Disease among Minnesota Business and Professional Men Followed Fifteen Years." *Circulation* XXXVIII (1963): 381-95.

7. Keys, Ancel and Francisco Grande. "Role of Dietary Fat in Human Nutrition III-Diet and the Epidemiology of Coronary Heart Disease." *Am J Public Health* 47 (1957): 1520-30.

8. Campbell, T. Colin and Thomas M. Campbell II. *The China Study*. Dallas: BenBella Books, 2006.

9. Pathway Genomics Newsroom. "Genetics loads the gun and environment pulls the trigger. – Dr. Francis Collins." Accessed on January 5, 2014. http://blog.pathway .com/genetics-loads-the-gun-and-environment-pulls-the-trigger-dr-francis-collins/.

10. Keys, Ancel. *Seven countries: a multivariate analysis of death and coronary heart disease*. Cambridge: Harvard University Press, 1980.

11. Blackburn, Henry. *Cardiovascular disease epidemiology*. Chapter 7. Accessed on November 18, 2013. http://www.epi.umn.edu/cvdepi/pdfs/07-Holland-Chap07copy.pdf.

12. Keys, Ancel and Margaret Keys. *Eat well and stay well (Revised edition)*. New York: Doubleday & Company, 1963.

13. Nestle, Marion. "Mediterranean diets: historical and research overview." *Am J Clin Nutr* 61(suppl): 1313S-20S

14. United States Department of Agriculture Center for Nutrition Policy and Promotion. "1980 Guidelines." Accessed November 28, 2013, http://www.cnpp.usda .gov/DGAs1980Guidelines.htm

15. Willett, Walter C., Frank Sacks, Antonia Trichopoulou, Greg Drescher, Anne Ferro-Luzzi, Elisabet Helsing, and Dimitrios Trichopoulos. "Mediterranean diet pyramid: a cultural model for healthy eating." *Am J Clin Nutr* 61 (1995): 1402S-6S.

16. Lewis, Barry, David R. Sullivan, and Gerald F. Watts. "Thought for food: Clinical evidence for the dietary prevention strategy in cardiovascular disease." *Int J Evid Based Healthc* 11 (2013): 330-36.

17. Hooper, Lee, Carolyn D. Summerbell, Rachel Thompson, Deidre Sills, Felicia G. Roberts, Helen J. Moore, and George Davey Smith. "Reduced or modified dietary fat for preventing cardiovascular disease." *The Cochrane Library* 5 (2012): 1-219.

18. Jacobs, David R., Linda C. Tapsell, and Normal J. Temple. "Food synergy: the key to balancing the nutrition research effort." *Public Health Reviews* 33, no.2 (2012): 507-29.

19. de Lorgeril, Michel, Patricia Salen, Jean-Louis Martin, Isabelle Monjaud, Jacques Delaye, and Nicole Mamelle. "Mediterranean diet, traditional risk factors, and the rate of cardiovascular complications after myocardial infarction: final report of the Lyon Diet Heart Study." *Circulation* 99 (1999): 779-85.

20. de Lorgeril Michel. "Mediterranean diet and cardiovascular disease: Historical perspective and latest evidence." *Curr Atheroscler Rep* 15 (2013): 370-4.

21. Estruch, Ramon, Emilio Ros, Jordi Salas-Salvado, Maria-Isabel Covas, Dolories Corella, Fernando Aros, Enrique Gomez-Gracia, Valentina Ruiz-Gutierrez, Miguel Fiol, Jose Lapetra, Rosa Maria Lamuela-Raventos, Lluis Serra-Majem, Xavier Pinto, Josep Basora, Miguel Angel Munoz, Jose V. Sorli, Jose Alfredo Martinez, and Miguel Angel Martinez-Gonzalez. "Primary prevention of cardiovascular disease with a Mediterranean diet." *N Engl J Med* 368, no. 14 (2013): 1279-90.

22. Salas-Salvado, Jordi, Monica Bullo, Ramon Estruch, Emilio Ros, Maria Isabel Covas, Nuria Ibarrola-Jurado, Dolores Corella, Fernando Aros, Enrique Gomez-Gracia, Valetina Ruiz-Gutierrez, Dora Romaguera, Jose Lapetra, Rosa Maria Lamuela-Raventos, Lluis Serra-Majem, Xavier Pinto, Josep Basora, Miguel Angel Munoz, Jose V. Sorli, and Miguel A. Martinez-Gonzalez. "Prevention of diabetes with Mediterranean diets: A subgroup analysis of a randomized trial." *Ann Intern Med* 160 (2014): 1-10.

23. Sofi, Francesco, Rosanna Abbate, Gian Franco Gensini, and Alessandro Casini. "Accruing evidence on benefits of adherence to the Mediterranean diet on health: an updated systematic review and meta-analysis. *Am J Clin Nutr* 92 (2010): 1189-96.

24. Trichopoulou, Antonia, Christina Bamia, Pagonia Lagiou, and Dimitrios Trichopoulos. "Conformity to traditional Mediterranean diet and breast cancer risk in the Greek EPIC (European Prospective Investigation into Cancer and Nutrition) cohort." *Am J Clin Nutr* 92 (2010): 620-5.

25. Psaltopoulou, Theodora, Theodoros N. Sergentanis, Demosthenes B. Panagiotakos, Ioannis N. Sergentanis, Rena Kosti. and Nikolaos Scarmeas. "Mediterranean diet and stroke, cognitive impairment, depression: A meta-analysis." *Ann Neurol* 74, no.4 (2013): 580-91.

26. Lourida, Ilianna, Maya Soni, Joanna Thompson-Coon, Nitin Purandare, Iain A. Lang, Obioha C. Ukoumunne, and David J. Llewellyn. "Mediterranean Diet, Cognitive Function, and Dementia: A Systematic Review." *Epidemiology* 24, no. 4 (2013): 479-89.

27. Esposito, Katherine, Raffaele Marfella, Miryam Ciotola, Carmen Di Palo, Francesco Giugliano, Giovanni Giugliano, Massimo D'Armiento, Francesco D'Andrea, and Dario Giugliano. "Effect of a Mediterranean-style diet on endothelial dysfunction and markers of vascular inflammation in the metabolic syndrome." *JAMA* 292, no.12 (2004): 1440-46.

28. Ruiz-Canela, Miguel, Ramon Estruch, Dolores Corella, Jordi Salas-Salvado, and Miguel A. Martinez-Gonzalez. "Association of Mediterranean diet with peripheral artery disease: the PREDIMED randomized trial." *JAMA* 311, no.4 (2014): 415-17.

29. Samieri, Cecilia, Qi Sun, Mary K. Townsend, Stephanie E. Chiuve, Olivia I. Okereke, Walter C. Willett, Meir Stampfer, and Francine Grodstein. "The Association Between Dietary Patterns at Midlife and Health in Aging: An Observational Study." *Ann Intern Med* 159, no. 9 (2013): 584-91.

CHAPTER 2

1. Milton, Katherine. "Hunter-gatherer diets-a different perspective." *Am J Cin Nutr* 71, no.3 (2000): 665-67.

2. Henry, Amanda G., Peter S. Unger, Benjamin H. Passey, Matt Sponhemier, Lloyd Rossouw, Marion Bamford, Paul Sandberg, Darryl J. de Ruiter, and Lee Berger. "The diet of Australopthecus sediba." *Nature* Accessed on January 30, 2014. http://www.nature.com/nature/journal/vaop/ncurrent/full/nature11185.html.

3. Wilford, John Noble. "Some prehumans feasted on bark instead of grasses." *New York Times*. Accessed January 29, 2014. http://www.nytimes.com/2012/06/28/science /australopithecus-sediba-preferred-forest-foods-fossil-teeth-suggest.html?_r=0.

4. Mercarder, J. "Mozambican grass seed consumption during the Middle Stone Age." *Science* 326, no. 5960 (2009): 1680-83.

5. Henry, Amanda. G., Alison. S. Brooks, and Dolores. R. Piperno. "Microfossils in calculus demonstrate consumption of plants and cooked foods in Neanderthal diets (Shanidar III, Iraq; Spy I and II, Belgium). *Proc Natl Acad Sci USA* Accessed online January 29, 2014. http://www.pnas.org/content/108/2/486.long.

6. Revedin, Anna, Biancamaria Aranguren, and Jiri Svoboda. "Thirty thousand-year-old evidence of plant food processing." *Proc Natl Acad Sci* 107, no. 44 (2010): 18815-19.

7. Barnard, Neal D. "Trends in food availability, 1909-2007." *Am J Clin Nutr* 91 (2010): 1530S-36S.

8. Orlich, Michael J., Pramil N. Singh, Joan Sabate, Karen Jaceldo-Siegl, Jing Fan, Synnove Knutsen, W. Lawrence Beeson, and Gary E. Fraser. "Vegetarian dietary patterns and mortality in Adventist Health Study 2." *JAMA Intern Med* 173, no. 13 (2013): 1230-38.

9. Huang, Tao, Bin Yang, Jusheng Zheng, Guipu Li, Mark L. Wahlqvist, and Duo Li. "Cardiovascular disease mortality and cancer incidence in vegetarians: a meta-analysis and systematic review." *Ann Nutr Metab* 60 (2013): 233-40.

10. Ferdowsian, Hope R., and Neal D. Barnard. "Effects of plant-based diets on plasma lipids." *Am J Cardiol* 104 (2009): 947-56.

11. Tuso, Philip J, Mohamed H. Ismail, Benjamin P. Ha, and Carole Bartolotto. "Nutritional update for physicians: plant-based diets." *Perm J* 17, no. 2 (2013): 61-66.

12, 13, 14. Uribarri, Jaime, Sandra Woodruff, Susan Goodman, Weijing Cai, Xue Chen, Renata Pyzik, Angie Young, Gary E. Striker, and Helen Vlassara. "Advanced glycation end products in foods and a practical guide to their reduction in the diet." *J Am Diet Assoc* 110, no. 6 (2010): 911-16.

15. Hedlund, Maria, Vered Padler-Karavani, Nissi M. Varki, and Ajit Varki. "Evidence for a human-specific mechanism for diet and antibody-mediated inflammation in carcinoma progression." *PNAS* 105, no. 48 (2008): 18936-41.

16. Koeth, Robert A., Zeneng Wang, Bruce S. Levison, Jennifer A. Buffa, Elin Org, Brendan T. Sheehy, Earl B. Britt, Xiaoming Fu, Yuping Wu, Lin Li, Jonathan D. Smith, Joseph A. DiDonato, Jun Chen, Hongzhe Li, Gary D. Wu, James D. Lewis, Manya Warrier, J. Mark Brown, Ronald M. Krauss, W. H. Wilson Tang, Frederic D. Bushman, Aldons J. Lusis, and Stanley L. Hazen. "Intestinal microbiota metabolism of L-carnitine, a nutrient found in red meat, promotes atherosclerosis." *Nature Medicine* 19 (2013): 578-85.

17. Ascherio, Alberto, Walter C. Willett, Eric B. Rimm, Edward L. Giovannucci, and Meir J. Stampfer. "Dietary iron intake and risk of coronary disease among men." *Circulation* 89 (1994): 969-74.

18. Qi, Lu, Rob M. van Dam, Kathryn Rexrode, and Frank B. Hu. "Heme iron from diet as a risk factor for coronary heart disease in women with type 2 diabetes." *Diabetes Care* 30 (2007): 101-06.

19. Grant, William B. "An ecological study of cancer mortality rates including indices for dietary iron and zinc." *Anticancer Research* 28 (2008): 1955-64.

20. National Institutes of Health Office of Dietary Supplements. "Iron Dietary Supplement Fact Sheet." Accessed on February 6, 2014. http://ods.od.nih.gov/fact sheets/Iron-HealthProfessional/#en79.

21. Oxford dictionary. Accessed February 3, 2014. http://www.oxforddictionaries .com/us/definition/american_english/synergy.

22. Pertea, Mihaela and Steven L. Salzberg. "Between a chicken and a grape: estimating the number of human genes." *Genome Bio* 11, no. 5 (2010): 206.

23. Jacobs, David R., Linda C. Tapsell, and Norman J. Temple. "Food synergy: the key to balancing the nutrition research effort." *Public Health Reviews* 33, no. 2 (2012): 507-29.

24. The Alpha-Tocopherol, Beta Carotene Cancer Prevention Study Group. "The effect of vitamin E and beta carotene on the incidence of lung cancer and other cancers in male smokers." *N Engl J Med* 330, no. 15 (1994): 1029-35.

25. Omenn, Gilbert S., Gary E. Goodman, Mark D. Thornquist, John Balmes, Mark R. Cullen, Andrew Glass, James P. Keogh, Frank L. Meyskens, Jr., Barbara Valanis, James H. Williams, Jr., Scott Barnhart, Martin G. Cherniack, Carl Andrew Brodkin, and Samuel Hammar. "Risk factors for lung cancer and for intervention effects in CARET, the beta-carotene and retinol efficacy trial." *J Natl Cancer Inst* 88 (1996): 1550-59.

26. Holick, Crystal N., Dominique S. Michaud, Rachael Stolzenberg-Solomon, Susan T. Mayne, Pirjo Pietinen, Philip R. Taylor, Jarmo Virtamo, and Demetrius Albanes. "Dietary carotenoids, serum β-carotene, and retinol and risk of lung cancer in the alpha-tocopherol, beta-carotene cohort study." *Am J Epidemiol* 156 (2002): 536-47.

27. Buettner, Dan. *The Blue Zones.* Washington D.C.: National Geographic Society, 2012.

28. Center for Disease Control and Prevention. "Smoking and Tobacco Use." Accessed on February 14, 2014. http://www.cdc.gov/tobacco/data_statistics/fact_sheets /health_effects/effects_cig_smoking/.

29. Supic, Gordana, Maja Jagodic, and Zvonko Magic. "Epigenetics: A new link between nutrition and cancer." *Nutrition and Cancer* 65, no. 6 (2013): 781-92.

30. Skiadas, P. K. and J. G. Lascaratos. "Dietetics in ancient Greek philosophy: Plato's concepts of healthy diet." *European J Clin Nutr* 55 (2001): 532-37.

31. Barnard, Neal D., Joshua Cohen, David J.A. Jenkins, Gabrielle Turner-McGrievy, Lisa Gloede, Amber Green, and Hope Ferdowsian. "A low-fat vegan diet and a conventional diabetes diet in the treatment of type 2 diabetes: a randomized, controlled, 74-wk clinical trial." *Am J Clin Nutr* 89 (2009): 1588S-96S.

32. Campbell, T. Colin and Thomas M. Campbell II. *The China Study.* Dallas: BenBella Books, 2006.

33. Academy of Nutrition and Dietetics. "Position of the Academy of Nutrition and Dietetics: Dietary fatty acids for healthy adults." *J Acad Nutr Diet* 114 (2014): 135-53.

34. Skiadas, PK and JG Lascaratos. "Dietetics in ancient Greek philosophy: Plato's concepts of healthy diet." *European Journal of Clinical Nutrition* 55 (2001): 533.

35. USDA. "US Nutrient Database." Accessed March 27, 2014, http://ndb.nal.usda .gov/.

36. Rizos, Evangelos C., Evangelia E. Ntzani, Eftychia Bika, and Moses S. Elisaf. "Association between omega-3 fatty acid supplementation and risk of major cardiovascular disease events: a systematic review and meta-analysis." *JAMA* 308, no. 10 (2012): 1024-33.

37. Kwak, Sang Mi, Seung-Kwon Myung, Young Jae Lee, and Hong Gwan Seo for the Korean Meta-Analysis Study Group. "Efficacy of omega-3 fatty acid supplements (eicosapentaenoic acid and docosahexaenoic acid) in the secondary prevention of cardiovascular disease: a meta-analysis of randomized, double-blind, placebo-controlled trials." *Arch Intern Med* 172, no. 9 (2012): 686-94.

38. Davis, Brenda and Vesanto Melina. *Becoming Vegan: Express Edition.* Summertown: Book Publishing Company, 2013.

39. Norris, Jack and Ginny Messina. "Omega-3 fatty acid recommendations for vegetarians." Accessed February 16, 2014. http://www.veganhealth.org/articles/omega3.

CHAPTER 4

1. Campbell, T. Colin, and Howard Jacobson. *Whole: Rethinking the Science of Nutrition.* Dallas: BenBella Books, 2013.

2. Campbell, T. Colin, and Howard Jacobson. *Whole: Rethinking the Science of Nutrition.* Dallas: BenBella Books, 2013, pages 285-86.

3. Campbell, T. Colin and Thomas M. Campbell II. *The China Study.* Dallas: BenBella Books, 2006.

4. U.S. Department of Agriculture. "USDA Nutrient Database for Standard Reference." Washington DC: U.S. Department of Agriculture, Agriculture Research Service, 2002. Accessed at http://www.nal.USDA.gov/fnic/foodcomp.

5. Holden, Joanne M., Alison L. Eldridge, Gary R. Beecher, Marilyn Buzzard, Seema Bhagwat, Carol S. Davis, Larry W. Douglass, Susan Gebhardt, David Haytowitz, and Sally Schakel. "Carotenoid content of U.S. foods: an update of the database." *Journal of Food Composition and Analysis* 12 (1999): 169-96.

6. Campbell, T. Colin and Thomas M. Campbell II. *The China Study*. Dallas: BenBella Books, 2006.

7. Kessler, David A. *The End of Overeating*. New York: Rodale, 2009.

8. World Health Organization. "Global Strategy on Diet, Physical Activity and Health." Accessed on February 25, 2014, http://www.who.int/dietphysicalactivity /fruit/en/index2.html.

9. Anderson, James W., Pat Baird, Richard H. Davis, Jr., Stefanie Ferreri, Mary Knudtson, Ashraf Koraym, Valerie Waters, and Christine L. Williams. "Health benefits of dietary fiber." *Nutrition Reviews* 67, no. 4 (2009): 188-205.

10. Linus Pauling Institute. "Fiber." Accessed on February 26, 2014, http://lpi .oregonstate.edu/infocenter/phytochemicals/fiber/.

11. American Institute for Cancer Research. "AICR's Foods that Fight Cancer: Soy." Accessed on February 26, 2014, http://www.aicr.org/foods-that-fight-cancer/soy .html.

12. American Institute on Cancer Research. "Soy." Accessed on March 1, 2014, http://www.aicr.org/foods-that-fight-cancer/soy.html#references.

13. Messina, Mark, and Gareth Redmond. "Effects of soy protein and soybean isoflavones on thyroid function in healthy adults and hypothyroid patients: a review of the relevant literature." *Thyroid* 16, no.3 (2006): 249-58.

14. Davis, Brenda and Vesanto Melina. *Becoming Vegan: Express Edition*. Summertown: Book Publishing Company, 2013.

15. Norris, Jack. "Omega-3 Fatty Acid Recommendations for Vegetarians." Accessed on March 1, 2014, http://veganhealth.org/articles/omega3#veganDHA.

16. Nestle, Marion, and Malden Nesheim. *Why Calories Count*. Berkeley: University of California Press, 2012.

17. Seguin, Rebecca, David M. Buchner, Jingmin Liu, Matthew Allison, Todd Manini, Ching-Yun Wang, JoAnn E. Manson, Catherine R. Messina, Mahesh J. Patel, Larry Moreland, Marcia L. Stefanick, and Andrea Z. LaCroix. "Sedentary behavior and mortality in older women: the women's health initiative." *Am J Preventive Med* 46, no. 2 (2014): 122-35.

CHAPTER 5

1. USDA. "National Nutrient Database for Standard Reference." Accessed March 6, 2014, http://ndb.nal.usda.gov/ndb/search/list.

2. The American Heart Association. "Fats and Oils: AHA Recommendation." Accessed on September 1, 2014, http://www.heart.org/HEARTORG/GettingHealthy /FatsAndOils/Fats101/Fats-and-Oils-AHA-Recommendation%5FUCM%5F31637 5%5FArticle.jsp

3. U.S. Food and Drug Administration. "FDA Targets Trans Fats in Processed Foods." Accessed on March 7, 2014, http://www.fda.gov/forconsumers/consumer updates/ucm372915.htm.

4. Linus Pauling Institute. "Phytosterols." Accessed on March 7, 2014, http://lpi .oregonstate.edu/infocenter/phytochemicals/sterols/.

5. Jenkins, Davis J. A., Cyril W. C. Kendall, Augustine Marchie, Dorothea A. Faulkner, Julia M. W. Wong, Russell de Souza, Azadeh Emam, Tina L. Parker, Edward Vidgen, Elke A. Trautwein, Karen G. Lapsley, Robert G. Josse, Lawrence A. Leiter, William Singer, and Philip W. Connelly. "Direct comparison of a dietary portfolio of cholesterol-lowering foods with a statin in hypercholesterolemic participants." *Am J Clin Nutr* 81 (2005): 380-87.

6. USDA. "Dietary Guidelines for Americans 2010." Accessed on March 8, 2014, http://www.health.gov/dietaryguidelines/dga2010/DietaryGuidelines2010.pdf.

7. Sabate, Joan, and Yen Ang. "Nuts and health outcomes: new epidemiologic evidence." *Am J Clin Nutr* 89 (2009): 1643S-48S.

8. Bes-Rastrollo, Maira, Nicole M. Wedick, Miguel Angel Martinez-Gonzalez, Tricia Y. Li, Laura Sampson, and Frank B. Hu. "Prospective study of nut consumption, long-term weight change, and obesity risk in women." *Am J Clin Nutr* 89 (2009): 1913-19.

CHAPTER 6

1. Tulchinsky, Theodore H. "Micronutrient deficiency conditions: global health issues." *Public Health Reviews* 32, no. 1 (2010): 243-55.

2. Mahan, L. Kathleen, & Sylvia Escott-Stump. *Krause's Food, Nutrition, & Diet Therapy, 11th Ed.* Philadelphia: Saunders, 2004.

3. National Institutes of Health Office of Dietary Supplements. "Vitamin B12 Fact Sheet for Consumers." Accessed on March 11, 2014, http://ods.od.nih.gov/factsheets /VitaminB12-QuickFacts/.

4. Food and Agricultural Organization Corporate Document Repository. "Chapter 5. B12." Accessed on March 11, 2014, http://www.fao.org/docrep/004/y2809e /y2809e0b.htm.

5. Norris, Jack. "Vitamin B12 Recommendations." Accessed on March 22, 2014, http://www.veganhealth.org/b12/rec.

6. Norman, Anthony W. "From vitamin D to hormone D: fundamentals of the vitamin D endocrine system essential for good health." *Am J Clin Nutr* 88 (2008): 491S-99S.

7. Lobo, Vijaya, A. Patil, A. Phatak, and N. Chandra. "Free radicals, antioxidants, and functional foods: impact on human health." *Pharmacogn Rev* 4, no. 8 (2010): 118-26.

8. Linus Pauling Institute Micronutrient Research Center for Optimum Health. "Vitamin C." Accessed on March 14, 2014, http://lpi.oregonstate.edu/infocenter /vitamins/vitaminC/.

9. Davis, Brenda, and Vesanto Melina. *Becoming Raw.* Summertown: Book Publishing Company, 2010.

10. David, Brenda, and Vesanto Melina. *Becoming Vegan Express Edition.* Summertown: Book Publishing Company, 2013.

11. Kerstetter, Jane E., Kimberly O. O'Brien, Donna M. Caseria, Diane E. Wall, and Karl L. Insogna. "The impact of dietary protein on calcium absorption and kinetic measures of bone turnover in women." *J Clin Endocrinol Metab* 90 (2005): 26-31.

12. National Institutes of Health Office of Dietary Supplements. "Iodine Fact Sheet for Health Professionals." Accessed on March 16, 2014, http://ods.od.nih.gov/fact sheets/Iodine-HealthProfessional/.

13. Linus Pauling Institute Micronutrient Research for Optimum Health. "Sodium (Chloride)." Accessed on March 17, 2014, http://lpi.oregonstate.edu/infocenter/minerals/sodium/.

14. Center for Disease Control and Prevention. "Americans consume too much sodium." Accessed on March 17, 2014, http://www.cdc.gov/features/dssodium/.

15. National Institutes of Health Office of Dietary Supplements. "Zinc Fact Sheet for Health Professionals." Accessed on March 17, 2014, http://ods.od.nih.gov/factsheets/Zinc-HealthProfessional/.

16. Guallar, Eliseo, Saverio Stranges, Cynthia Mulrow, Lawrence J. Appel, and Edgar R. Miller III. "Enough is Enough: Stop Wasting Money on Vitamin and Mineral Supplements." *Ann Intern Med* 159, no. 12 (2013): 850-51.

17. U.S. Food and Drug Administration. "Current Good Manufacturing Practices (CGMPs) for Dietary Supplements." Accessed on March 22, 2014, http://www.fda.gov/Food/GuidanceRegulation/CGMP/ucm079496.htm.

18. Kimpimaki, T., M. Erkkola, S. Korhonen, A. Kupila, S.M. Virtanen, J. Ilonen, O. Simell, and M. Knip. "Short-term exclusive breastfeeding predisposes young children with increased genetic risk of type 1 diabetes to progressive beta-cell autoimmunity." *Diabetologia* 44 (2001): 63-69.

19. Saukkonen, T., S. M. Virtanen, M. Karppinen, H. Reijonen, J. Ilonen, L. Rasanen, H. K. Akerblom, and E. Savilahti. "Significance of cow's milk protein antibodies as risk factor for childhood IDDM: interactions with dietary cow's milk intake and HLA-DQB1 genotype. Childhood diabetes in Finland study group." *Diabetologia* 41, no. 1 (1998): 72-78.

20. Sampson, Hugh A. "Food allergy. Part 1: Immunopathogenesis and clinical disorders." *J Allergy Clin Immunol* 103 (1999): 717-28.

21. Buettner, Dan. *The Blue Zones, Second Edition: 9 Lessons for Living Longer From the People Who've Lived the Longest.* Washington, D.C.: National Geographic Society, 2012.

22. Academy of Nutrition and Dietetics, Dietitians of Canada, and American College of Sports Medicine. "Nutrition and athletic performance." *Medicine and Science in Sports and Exercise* 41, no. 3 (2009): 709-31.

CHAPTER 7

1. Rosenbaum, Michael, and Rudolph L. Leibel. "Adaptive thermogenesis in humans." *Int J Obes (Lond)* 34, no. 1 (2010): S47-S55.

2. http://www.happycow.net/

CHAPTER 9

1. U.S. Dry Bean Council. "Pre-Prep." Accessed on March 8, 2014, http://www.usdrybeans.com/recipes/beans-pre-prep/.

NUTRIENTS CHARTS AND TABLES

1. Institute of Medicine. "Dietary Reference Intakes Tables and Applications." Accessed on July 11, 2014, http://www.iom.edu/Activities/Nutrition/SummaryDRIs/DRI-Tables.aspx

Index

Academy of Nutrition and Dietetics (AND), 30, 32

ACHIEVE (Affirmative Convenient Habitual Infinitesimal Effortless Victorious Exact), 156–158

Advanced glycation end products (AGEs), 20

Affirmative Convenient Habitual Infinitesimal Effortless Victorious Exact. *See* ACHIEVE

AGEs. *See* Advanced glycation end products

Aioli, 221–222

ALA. *See* Alpha-linolenic acid

Alcohol consumption, 34–35, 91 (fig.), 93 (fig.), 108

Alcoholism, 119, 121, 129

Allbaugh, Leland, 6, 36

Almonds
   Almond Sun-Dried Tomato Hummus, 193
   Basic Nut Milk, 176, 185
   DIY Nut Butter, 185–186
   Ganache Parfait with Poached Berries, 237–238

Alpha-linolenic acid (ALA), 36, 37, 38, 77 (table)

Alpha-tocopherol, 116–117

Amaretto Gelato, 238–239

Amino acids
   in legumes, 73
   metabolism of, 121–122
   in nuts, 106
   role of, 94 (table)
   types of, 96

AND. *See* Academy of Nutrition and Dietetics

Animal foods
   antibiotics in, 19
   cancer and, 18, 20
   compassion and, 57–59
   in Cretan diet, 7–8, 16–17, 36
   disease and, 18–20
   environmental impact of, 45–49
   factory farming of, 57–59
   fats in, 36–38, 98, 99
   in food pyramids, 90 (fig.)
   growth hormones in, 18–19
   iron in, 20–21
   overconsumption of, x–xi, 7–8, 17, 44–45
   plant nutrients compared to, 64–65, 64 (table)
   protein in, 64 (table), 96
   psychology of eating, 49–56
   toxins in, 19–20, 36–38, 44

Antibiotics, 19

Antioxidants, 116–117, 120

Antipasti. See Small plates

Appliances, 167–169

Apricots
   grilled, 238–239
   paste, 196

Arugula, 220–221

Asia
   China Study, 10, 29, 64
   flavors, 92
   Japanese diet, 9–10, 27–28, 29

Athletes
   post-training meals, 138–139, 155–156
   Vegiterranean Athlete's Drink, 190–191

Avocado
   benefits of, 107
   fatty acids in, 77 (table)
   Smoky Avocado Dip, 194

Baba Ganoush, 192

Baby food, 134–135

Bacteria, gut, 72, 130
Bakeware, 169
Baking
    Baked Oat Bread, 215–216
    egg-free, 177–178
    oil-free, 180
Banana Sandwich, 217–218
Barnard, Neal D., vii–viii, 17, 29
Basic Nut or Seed Milk, 176, 185
Basil
    Basil Aioli, 221–222
    Easy Caprese, 199–200
    Lemon Basil Dressing, 196–197
    Tempeh Cutlet Sandwich with Arugula
        and Basil Aioli, 220–221
Baur, Gene, 57–59
Beans
    benefits of, 73–75
    Dilled Rice with Lima Beans, 201–202
    prepping and cooking, 103, 187–188
    protein in, 97 (table)
    sprouting, 188
    storage of, 103, 173
    See also Cannellini beans; Chickpeas; Ful;
        Soy
Belila, 222–223
Bell peppers. See Red bell peppers
Berries
    Brain-Boosting Blue Smoothie, 189
    Ganache Parfait with Poached Berries,
        237–238
    Summer Fruit Tart, 236
Beta-carotene, 23–24
Betta' than Feta, 183
Bettermilk, 183–184
Beverages
    Basic Nut or Seed Milk, 176, 185
    coffee, 126
    meal plan choices for, 150
    Moroccan Mint Chia Tea, 189–190
    tea, 100, 126, 189–191
    Vegiterranean Athlete's Drink, 190–191
    water, 93 (fig.), 100, 139
    See also Smoothies
Bhamia (Okra), 211–212
Biotin, 121
Bisphenol A (BPA), 103
Blenders, 168
Blood flow, 106, 117–118
BPA. See Bisphenol A
Brain-Boosting Blue Smoothie, 189
Brazil nuts, 128

Breads
    Baked Oat Bread, 215–216
    Carrot Muffins, 217
    in food pyramids, 90 (fig.), 91 (fig.), 93
        (fig.)
    protein in, 97 (table)
    Stone-Ground Cornbread, 216–217
Breakfast
    Breakfast Sunshine Salad, 206–207
    meal plans, 146–147, 153
Broad beans. See Ful
Broccoli
    Cheesy Smoky Butternut Squash Pasta,
        224–225
    fatty acids in, 77 (table)
    protein in, 97 (table)
Broth, 179
Buffet-style meals, 143, 164
Bulgur, 208–209
Buttermilk. See Bettermilk
Butternut squash, 70 (table), 117 (table)
    Cheesy Smoky Butternut Squash Pasta,
        224–225
    Couscous Soup, 212–213

Cabbage, 204–205
Caesar dressing, 195
Caffeine, 151
Calciferol, 113–114
Calcium, 113, 123–124
Calories
    animal and plant comparison of, 64–65, 64
        (table)
    CCC tenet on, 80–83
    increase in, 33–34, 134
    reduction in, 9, 27–28, 80–83
Campbell, T. Colin, 10, 29, 63
Cancer
    animal foods and, 18, 20
    mortality rates, 5, 29
    plant foods and, vii, 23–24, 69, 74, 75
Cannellini beans
    Cilantro Lime Dressing, 197
    Hummus of the Earth, 192–193
    Lemon Basil Dressing, 196–197
    White Bean and Rosemary Dip, 194
Caprese, 199–200
Carbohydrates, 93–95
    See also Fruit; Grains; Legumes; Starch;
        Vegetables
Cardiovascular disease (CVD), 4–5, 8–11,
    13–14, 29

Carnism, 53–56
Carotenoids, 22, 23–24, 116, 117 (table)
Carrots
  Breakfast Sunshine Salad, 206–207
  Carrot Muffins, 217
  Savory Veggie Pancakes, 218
Cashews
  Amaretto Gelato, 238–239
  Basic Nut Milk, 185
  Cashew Caesar Dressing, 195
  DIY Nut Butter, 185–186
Cautious Calorie Consciousness (CCC),
  80–83
Cereal
  Belila, 222–223
  Chocolate Crispy Fruit Squares, 239–240
  for infants, 135
Champagne Vinaigrette, Peach, 195–196
Chard, 201
Cheese substitutions, 176–177
  Betta' than Feta, 183
  Cheesy Smoky Butternut Squash Pasta,
    224–225
  Parma Shake, 182
  Savory Sprinkles, 182–183
Chemicals. See Phytochemicals; Toxins
Chia seeds, 106
  Chocolate Hazelnut Chia Pudding, 234
  egg replacement with, 177–178
  fatty acids in, 77–78
  Moroccan Mint Chia Tea, 189–190
Chickpeas
  Couscous Soup, 212–213
  Falafel, 225–226
  Lemon Chard with Chickpeas, 201
  protein in, 97 (table)
  Quinoa and Chickpea Tabbouleh Salad,
    208–209
  Tuscan Garden Salad, 209–210
  See also Hummus
Children
  Banana Sandwich for, 217–218
  Chocolate Crispy Fruit Squares for,
    239–240
  Vegiterranean Diet for, 135–137
  Vegiterranean Meal Plan for, 154–155
China Study, 10, 29, 64
Chips, 198–199
Chloe's Kitchen (Coscarelli), 200
Chlorophyll, 75
Chocolate
  Banana Sandwich, 217–218

Chocolate Crispy Fruit Squares, 239–240
Chocolate Hazelnut Chia Pudding, 234
  Ganache Parfait with Poached Berries,
    237–238
Cholesterol
  CVD connection to, 8–10
  improving, 32, 76, 98, 120
  properties of, 99
Choline, 122
Chowder, 214
Cilantro Lime Dressing, 197
Cobalamin, 111–112, 113 (table)
Coconut, 107
  Amaretto Gelato, 238–239
  Breakfast Sunshine Salad, 206–207
  milk, 176
  Vegiterranean Athlete's Drink, 190–191
Coenzymes, 119
Coffee, 126
Comfortably Unaware (Oppenlander), 45
Community Supported Agriculture (CSA),
  102
Compassion, 57–59
The Complete Idiot's Guide to Plant-Based
  Nutrition (Hever), 52, 132
Condimenti per Insalata. See Dressings
Condiments, 108, 151, 172, 174
Cookies, 235
Cooking
  beans, 103, 187–188
  leafy greens, 75–76
  lentils, 103, 186–187
  oil-free, 34, 107, 179–180
  simplicity and, 67
  thickeners, 106, 179
  See also Baking; Kitchen
Cookware, 169
Corn
  Cornbread, 216–217
  Polenta with Mushroom Ragu, 231–232
  Potato Corn Chowder, 214
Coscarelli, Chloe, 200
Couscous Soup, 212–213
Cravings, 66–67, 78, 79, 145
Cretan diet, 6–8, 16–17, 36
CSA. See Community Supported Agriculture
CVD. See Cardiovascular disease

Dairy
  politics of, 43
  substitutions, 176–177, 182–185, 224–225
Date Paste, 184

Davis, Brenda, 77
Dehydrators, 168–169
Delicious Dolmas, 203
Desserts
  Chocolate Crispy Fruit Squares, 239–240
  Chocolate Hazelnut Chia Pudding, 234
  in Cretan diet, 7
  frozen, 179, 238–239
  Ganache Parfait with Poached Berries,
    237–238
  Grilled Nectarines with Amaretto Gelato,
    238–239
  Italian Wedding Cookies, 235
  meal plan choices for, 150
  Summer Fruit Tart, 236
DHA. *See* Docosahexaenoic acid
Diabetes, 14, 18, 20, 35, 78, 95
Diet
  CVD and, 4–5, 8–11, 13–14, 29
  epigenetics and, 26–27
  fad, 24, 62
  as health and longevity factor, vii, 25–26
  Japanese, 9–10, 27–28, 29
  politics of, 43–44
  protein, 96
  pyramids, 11–12, 89–93, 90 (fig.), 91 (fig.),
    93 (fig.), 100–108
  research challenges, 12–13
  See also Mediterranean diet; Plant-based
    diet; Vegiterranean Diet
Diet for a New America (Robbins), 49
Dietary Guidelines for Americans, 11
Dietitians, 43, 51–52
Digestive problems. *See* Gastrointestinal
  problems
Dilled Rice with Lima Beans, 201–202
Dining out
  parties and potlucks, 163–164
  restaurants, 161–163
  traveling, 164–166
Dinner meal plans, 148–149, 154
Dionysus, 34–35
Dips. *See* Sauces and spreads
Diseases
  animal foods and, 18–20
  cardiovascular, 4–5, 8–11, 13–14, 29
  Crete and United States comparison of,
    7–8
  diabetes, 14, 18, 20, 35, 78, 95
  historical shift in, 4–5
  kidney, 76, 128, 129
  Mediterranean diet and, 13–14

  obesity-related, 27, 33–34
  smoking-related, 26
  sweeteners and, 78
  thyroid, 74, 125
  See also Cancer; Gastrointestinal problems
DIY Nut or Seed Butter, 185–186
Docosahexaenoic acid (DHA), 37, 38
Dolci. See Desserts
Dolmas, 203–204
Dressings
  Basil Aioli, 221–222
  Cashew Caesar Dressing, 195
  Cilantro Lime Dressing, 197
  Fresh Tomato Dressing, 209–210
  Lemon Basil Dressing, 196–197
  Peach Champagne Vinaigrette, 195–196
  seeds for, 106
  Tahina, 191

Easy Caprese, 199–200
Eat Well and Stay Well (Keys), 11
Eating out. *See* Dining out
Egg substitutions, 177–178
  Basil Aioli, 221–222
  Shakshuka (Middle Eastern Tofu Scramble),
    223–224
Eggplant
  Baba Ganoush, 192
  Moussaka, 232–233
  Red Hot Eggplant Salad, 210–211
  Roasted Vegetable Sandwich Rolls, 219
  Simple Roasted Vegetables, 202–203
Eicosapentaenoic acid (EPA), 37, 38
Electrolytes, 127, 139
Emotional eating, 83, 140–141
Energy bars, 239–240
Environment
  animal foods impact on, 45–49
  epigenetics and, 26–27
  free radicals, 117
EPA. *See* Eicosapentaenoic acid
EPIC. *See* European Prospective Investigation
  into Cancer and Nutrition
Epigenetics, 26–27
European Prospective Investigation into
  Cancer and Nutrition (EPIC), vii
Exercise, 25–26, 83–85, 100
  See also Athletes

Factory farming, 57–59
Fad diets, 24, 62
Falafel, 225–226

Farm Sanctuary, 57, 59
Fassulia (Green Beans) and Potatoes,
    229–230
Fats, 76–78, 97–100
  in animal foods, 36–38, 98, 99
  benefits of, 29–30, 76–78, 98, 105–107
  CVD and, 8–10
  in fish, 36–38
  in food pyramids, 90 (fig.), 91 (fig.), 93
    (fig.), 105–107
  hydrogenated, 30, 31–32, 98–99
  monounsaturated, 31–32, 98
  oil-free cooking, 34, 107, 179–180
  olive oil, 28–34, 77 (table)
  omega fatty acids, 30, 36–38, 77–78, 77
    (table), 98
  phytosterol, 99
  polyunsaturated, 30, 31–32, 36–38, 98
  saturated, 30, 32, 98
  synergy with, 22, 24
  trans, 30, 31–32, 98–99
  weight loss and, 76, 106
Fava beans. *See Ful*
Feta, 183
Fiber, 71–73
Fish, 36–38
Flavors
  cheesy, 177
  condiments, 108, 151, 172, 174
  ethnic interchangeability of, x, 92, 172
  of hyper-palatable foods, 66, 82, 140
  of Mediterranean, xi, 28, 108
  for oil-free cooking, 180
Flaxseeds, 106
  egg replacement with, 177
  fatty acids in, 77 (table)
  milk, 176
  protein in, 97 (table)
Folate, 121–122
Food addiction, 66–67, 78, 79, 145
Food journals, 159
Food processors, 168
Food pyramids. *See* Pyramids
Food synergy. *See* Synergy
Free radicals, 117
Freezer staples, 160, 174–175
Fresh Tomato Dressing, 209–210
Frozen desserts, 179, 238–239
Fruit
  Chocolate Crispy Fruit Squares, 239–240
  consumption increase in, 101–102
  dried, 168–169, 172

egg replacement with, 178
fiber in, 72–73
in food pyramids, 90 (fig.), 91 (fig.), 93
    (fig.), 100–102
juicing, 168
oil replacement with, 180
phytochemicals in, 68–69, 70 (table)
selecting, 102
Summer Fruit Tart, 236
See also specific types of fruit
Ful (crushed fava bean dish)
  Green, 226–227
  Medames, 227–228

Gadgets, 170–171
Ganache Parfait with Poached Berries,
    237–238
Gardening, 102
Gastrointestinal problems
  beans and, 187
  fiber and, 71–72, 73
  Hever's history of, 41, 51
  probiotics for, 130
  vitamin B12 deficiency and, 111
Gelato, 238–239
Genetically modified organisms (GMOs), 75
Genetics, 9–10, 26–27
Gluten-free
  Baked Oat Bread, 215–216
  Belila, 222–223
  grains, 104, 171
  Tabbouleh, 208–209
Glycemic index, 95
N-glycolylneuraminic acid (Neu5Gc), 20
GMOs. *See* Genetically modified organisms
Goals and habits
  setting, 156–158
  tools for achieving, 158–166
Goitrogens, 125
Government subsidies, 43–44
Grains
  enriched, 104
  fiber in, 73
  in food pyramids, 90 (fig.), 91 (fig.), 93
    (fig.), 103–105
  gluten-free, 104, 171
  protein in, 97 (table)
  refined, 104
  sprouted, 105
  storage for, 173
  See also specific types of grains
Green Beans and Potatoes, 229–230

Green *Ful*, 226–227
Green smoothies, 126–127, 139, 190
Greens. *See* Leafy greens
Greger, Michael, 32
Grilling
    animal foods, toxins in, 19
    Grilled Nectarines with Amaretto Gelato, 238–239

Habits. *See* Goals and habits
Hatz Lentil Soup, 213–214
Hazelnuts, 234
HCAs. *See* Heterocyclic amines
Health and longevity
    factors, vii, 25–26
    goals and habits for, 156–166
Hearty Red Lentil Stew, 230–231
Hempseeds, 77 (table), 106
    Basic Seed Milk, 176, 185
    DIY Seed Butter, 185–186
    Savory Sprinkles, 182–183
Herbs, 108, 151, 172, 174
    See also Flavors; *specific types of herbs*
Heterocyclic amines (HCAs), 19–20
Hever, Julieanna
    books by, 52, 132
    gastrointestinal problems for, 41, 51
    inspirations of, ix–xi, 49–52, 57
Hippocrates, 4
Hormones
    in animal food, 18–19
    cholesterol and, 99
    in soy, 74
    stress, 26
Hot, Sweet, and Sour *Bhamia* (Okra), 211–212
Hummus
    Almond Sun-Dried Tomato Hummus, 193
    Hummus of the Earth, 192–193
    Potato Cups, 200–201
Hunger
    malnutrition, 45, 47, 110–111
    tracking satiety and, 81–82, 137, 159
Hydrogenated fats, 30, 31–32, 98–99
Hyper-palatable foods, 66, 82, 140

Ice cream, 179, 238–239
IGF-1. *See* Insulin-like growth factor 1
Infants, 134–135
Insalata. See Salads
Insulin-like growth factor 1 (IGF-1), 18–19
Iodine, 125–126

Iron, 126–127
    for infants, 135
    for pregnancy, 133
    sources and absorption of, 20–21, 201
Isoflavones, 74
Israeli Salad, 207–208
Italian-inspired dishes, ix, xi
    Basil Aioli, 221–222
    Easy Caprese, 199–200
    Grilled Nectarines with Amaretto Gelato, 238–239
    Italian Wedding Cookies, 235
    Polenta with Mushroom Ragu, 231–232

Japanese diet, 9–10, 27–28, 29
Journals, 159
Joy, Melanie, 52–56
Juicers, 168

Kale
    Brain-Boosting Blue Smoothie, 189
    carotenoids in, 117 (table)
    fatty acids in, 77 (table)
    protein in, 97 (table)
    Sunrise Kale Chips, 198–199
Keys, Ancel, 8–12
Kids. *See* Children
Kitchen
    appliances, 167–169
    freezer staples, 160, 174–175
    gadgets, 170–171
    pantry staples, 160, 171–174
    refrigerator staples, 160, 174, 182–186
    storage, 103, 170, 173–174
    utensils, 169–170
Knives, 170

Labels, 25, 62–63, 99
Laron syndrome, 18
Latin American flavors, 92
Leafy greens
    benefits of, 75–76
    calcium inhibitors in, 124
    fatty acids in, 77 (table)
    in food pyramids, 90 (fig.), 91 (fig.), 93 (fig.)
    Lemon Chard with Chickpeas, 201
    protein in, 97 (table)
    in smoothies, 126–127, 139, 189, 190
    See also Kale; Spinach
Leftovers, 145, 175
Legumes
    benefits of, 73–75

in food pyramids, 90 (fig.), 91 (fig.), 93 (fig.), 102–103
    See also Beans; Lentils
Lemon
    Lemon Basil Dressing, 196–197
    Lemon Chard with Chickpeas, 201
    zesting and juicing, 181
Lentils
    benefits of, 73–75
    Hatz Lentil Soup, 213–214
    Hearty Red Lentil Stew, 230–231
    Moussaka, 232–233
    Mujadara, 228–229
    prepping and cooking, 103, 186–187
    protein in, 97 (table)
    sprouting, 188
Lifestyle
    CVD and, 8–11
    epigenetics and, 26–27
    Mediterranean, 6, 24–26
Lima beans, 201–202
Lime dressing, 197
Lists, 158–159
Longevity. See Health and longevity
Lunch meal plans, 147–148, 154
Lyon Diet Heart Study, 13–14

Macronutrients, 94 (table)
    See also Carbohydrates; Fats; Protein
Magnesium, 127
Main dishes
    Belila, 222–223
    Cheesy Smoky Butternut Squash Pasta, 224–225
    Falafel, 225–226
    Fassulia (Green Beans) and Potatoes, 229–230
    Ful Medames, 227–228
    Green Ful, 226–227
    Hearty Red Lentil Stew, 230–231
    Moussaka, 232–233
    Mujadara, 228–229
    Polenta with Mushroom Ragu, 231–232
    Shakshuka (Middle Eastern Tofu Scramble), 223–224
Malnutrition, 45, 47, 110–111
Meal planning. See Vegiterranean Meal Plan
Measurements, 81
Meats, mock, 178–179
    See also Animal foods
Mediterranean diet
    calorie reduction in, 27–28

Cretan, 6–8, 16–17, 36
disease and, 13–14
ethnic interchangeability of, x, 92, 172
flavors of, xi, 28, 108
foods in, vii, 5–6, 7, 89, 90 (fig.)
history of, 3–4, 6–8
as lifestyle, 6, 24–26
myths of, 28–38
pyramid, 11–12, 89, 90 (fig.)
research, vii, 13–14
synergy of, 22–24, 62, 72
    See also Plant-based diet
Mexican Wedding Cookies, 235
Microalgae, 131, 133
Micronutrients. See Minerals; Vitamins
Middle Eastern Tofu Scramble, 223–224
Milk, 176
    Basic Nut or Seed Milk, 176, 185
    Bettermilk, 183–184
    breast, 97, 134
Mindfulness, 85–86
    See also Cautious Calorie Consciousness
Minerals
    inhibitors, 75–76, 124, 125
    major types of, 123–129
    overview, 110, 123
    See also Supplements
Minnesota Business and Professional Men's Study, 9
Mint tea, 189–190
Monounsaturated fats (MUFAs), 31–32, 98
Moroccan Mint Chia Tea, 189–190
Mortality rates, 5, 7–8, 25–26, 29, 83
Motivation, 156
Moussaka, 232–233
Movement, 25–26, 83–85, 100
    See also Athletes
MUFAs. See Monounsaturated fats
Muffins, 217
Mujadara, 228–229
Mushrooms
    as meat replacer, 179
    Moussaka, 232–233
    Polenta with Mushroom Ragu, 231–232
Myths
    fish, 36–38
    olive oil, 28–34
    red wine, 34–35

Nectarines, 238–239
Nestle, Marion, 11
Neu5Gc. See N-glycolylneuraminic acid

Neurological disorders, 111, 119, 125
Nhat Hanh, Thich, 86
Niacin, 120
Noritos, 148
Nutrients
    animal and plant comparison of, 64–65, 64
        (table)
    essential, 68
    See also Carbohydrates; Fats; Protein
Nutrition school, 43, 51–52
Nutritional yeast, 172
    See also Cheese substitutions
Nutritionism, 62–63
Nuts
    Banana Sandwich, 217–218
    Basic Nut Milk, 176, 185
    benefits of, 105–106
    DIY Nut Butter, 185–186
    fatty acids in, 77 (table)
    fiber in, 73
    Parma Shake, 182
    protein in, 97 (table)
    storage of, 173–174
    See also specific types of nuts

Oats
    Baked Oat Bread, 215–216
    milk, 176
Obesity, 27, 33–34
Oil
    cutting out, 34, 107, 179–180
    olive, 28–34, 77 (table)
Okinawan Japanese diet, 27–28, 29
Okra, 211–212
Olive oil, 28–34, 77 (table)
Olives
    benefits of, 31 (table), 33, 107
    Tuscan Garden Salad, 209–210
Omega fatty acids, 30, 36–38, 77–78, 77
    (table), 98
Oppenlander, Richard, 45–49
Organic produce, 19, 75
Overeating, 27–28
Oxalates, 75–76, 124

Packaging, 62–65
PAHs. *See* Polycyclic aromatic hydrocarbons
Pancakes, 218
Pane. See Breads
Panini. See Sandwiches
Pantothenic acid, 120–121
Pantry staples, 160, 171–174

Parfait, 237–238
Parma Shake, 182
Passey, Benjamin H., 16
Pasta
    Cheesy Smoky Butternut Squash Pasta,
        224–225
    in food pyramids, 90 (fig.), 91 (fig.), 93
        (fig.)
    Primavera, 149
    protein in, 97 (table)
Peaches
    grilled, 238–239
    Peach Champagne Vinaigrette, 195–196
Peanuts, 103
Peas. *See* Legumes
Phytates, 124, 129
Phytochemicals, 33, 35, 68–69, 70 (table)
Phytoestrogens, 74
Phytosterols, 99
Piatti principali. See Main dishes
Planning. *See* Prepping; Vegiterranean Meal
    Plan
Plant-based diet
    AGEs in, 20
    ancestry and, 16
    ancient philosophy on, 4
    animal nutrients comparison to, 64–65, 64
        (table)
    benefits of, 17–18, 69
    cancer reduction in, vii, 23–24, 69, 74, 75
    carnism ideology and, 53–56
    definition of, 17
    fatty acids in, 36, 37, 77–78, 77 (table), 98
    fiber in, 71–73
    Hever's start in, 49–52, 57
    iron in, 20–21
    leafy green importance in, 75–76
    legume importance in, 73–75, 102–103
    minerals found in, 123–129
    phytochemicals in, 33, 35, 68–69, 70 (table)
    phytoestrogens in, 74
    phytosterols in, 99
    protein in, 64 (table), 97 (table)
    pyramid, 89, 90 (fig.), 91–92
    raw, 29
    substitutions, 175–180
    synergy of, 22–24, 62, 72
Plastic, 103
Plato, 4, 30, 35
Polenta with Mushroom Ragu, 231–232
Polycyclic aromatic hydrocarbons (PAHs),
    19–20

Polyunsaturated fats (PUFAs), 30, 31–32, 36–38, 98
Potassium, 127–128
Potatoes
    Fassulia (Green Beans) and Potatoes, 229–230
    Potato Corn Chowder, 214
    Potato Cups, 200–201
Potlucks, 163–164
Prebiotics, 72
PREDIMED (*Prevencion con Dieta Mediterranea*), 13–14
Pregnancy, 132–133
Prepping, 160
    beans, 103, 187–188
    lentils, 103, 186–187
Pressure cookers, 168
Prevencion con Dieta Mediterranea. See PREDIMED
Probiotics, 130
Processed foods
    complexity of, 65–66
    craving, 66–67, 78, 79, 145
    grains, refined, as, 104
    hyper-palatable foods, 66, 82, 140
    labels on, 25, 62–63, 99
    omitting, 44–45
    problems with, x–xi, 24, 25, 42
    sodium in, 128–129
    soy-based, 74–75
    trans fats as, 98–99
    whole foods compared to, 21–22
Produce
    organic, 19, 75
    seasonal, freezing, 175
    selecting, viii, 102
    See also Fruit; Vegetables
Protagoras, 30
Protein
    animal sources of, 64, 96
    for athletes, 139
    diet high in, 96
    plant sources of, 64, 64 (table), 97 (table)
    role and benefits of, 95–97
    for seniors, 138
    See also Amino acids
Pudding, 234
PUFAs. *See* Polyunsaturated fats
Pumpkin Pie Green Smoothie, 190
Pyramids
    Mediterranean, 11–12, 89, 90 (fig.)
    plant-based, 89, 90 (fig.), 91–92

Vegiterranean, 91 (fig.), 92–93, 93 (fig.), 100–108
Pyridoxine, 121

Quinoa
    Belila, 222–223
    protein in, 97 (table)
    Quinoa and Chickpea Tabbouleh Salad, 208–209

Ragu, 231–232
Rainbow
    eating colors of, 68–69, 70 (table)
    Rainbow Stuffed Cabbage Rolls, 204–205
Raw foodists, 29
Recommended Dietary Allowance (RDA)
    for carbohydrates, 95
    for fatty acids, 38, 77–78, 77 (table)
    for fiber, 71
    for fruit and vegetables, 101
    for protein, 97
    for vitamin B12, 112, 113 (table)
Red bell peppers
    Israeli Salad, 207–208
    Roasted Vegetable Sandwich Rolls, 219
    Savory Veggie Pancakes, 218
    Simple Roasted Vegetables, 202–203
Red Hot Eggplant Salad, 210–211
Refrigerator staples, 160, 174, 182–186
Restaurant menus, 161–163
Riboflavin, 119–120
Rice
    cookers/steamers, 168
    Delicious Dolmas, 203–204
    Dilled Rice with Lima Beans, 201–202
    Mujadara, 228–229
    protein in, 97 (table)
    Rainbow Stuffed Cabbage Rolls, 204–205
Roasted Vegetables
    Roasted Vegetable Sandwich Rolls, 219
    Simple Roasted Vegetables, 202–203
Robbins, John, 49
Robertson, Robin, 181, 209–210, 235
Rockefeller Foundation, 6
Rosemary, 194
Russian Tea Cookies, 235

Salad dressings. *See* Dressings
Salads
    Breakfast Sunshine Salad, 206–207
    Israeli Salad, 207–208

Salads (*continued*)
Quinoa and Chickpea Tabbouleh Salad,
208–209
Red Hot Eggplant Salad, 210–211
Tabbouleh, 208–209
Tuscan Garden Salad, 209–210
Salse. See Sauces and spreads
Salt, 125–126
Sandwiches
Banana Sandwich, 217–218
Roasted Vegetable Sandwich Rolls, 219
Tempeh Cutlet Sandwich with Arugula
and Basil Aioli, 220–221
Sarno, Chad, 181, 195–196, 220–221, 237–239
Satiety, 28, 81–82, 137, 159
Saturated fats (SFAs), 30, 32, 98
Sauces and spreads
Almond Sun-Dried Tomato Hummus, 193
Baba Ganoush, 192
Cashew Caesar Dressing, 195
Hummus of the Earth, 192–193
for Moussaka, 233
seed thickeners for, 106
Smoky Avocado Dip, 194
Sofrito, 24, 197–198
Tahina, 191
White Bean and Rosemary Dip, 194
Savory Sprinkles, 182–183
Savory Veggie Pancakes, 218
Schedules, 159–160
Scramble, 223–224
Seasoning. *See* Flavors
Seeds
Banana Sandwich, 217–218
Basic Seed Milk, 176, 185
DIY Seed Butter, 185–186
fatty acids in, 77 (table), 78
fiber in, 73
as thickeners, 106
See also Chia seeds; Flaxseeds; Hempseeds;
Sunflower seeds
Seitan, 179
Selenium, 125, 128
Seniors, 137–138
Seven Countries Study, 9, 10, 29
SFAs. *See* Saturated fats
Shakshuka (Middle Eastern Tofu Scramble),
223–224
Shopping lists, 158
Simple Roasted Vegetables, 202–203
Simplicity, 65–67
Skin problems, 120, 121

Slow cookers, 168
Small plates
Delicious Dolmas, 203
Dilled Rice with Lima Beans, 201–202
Easy Caprese, 199–200
Lemon Chard with Chickpeas, 201
Potato Cups, 200–201
Rainbow Stuffed Cabbage Rolls, 204–205
Simple Roasted Vegetables, 202–203
Sunrise Kale Chips, 198–199
Smoking, 26
Smoky Avocado Dip, 194
Smoothies, 126–127, 139
Brain-Boosting Blue Smoothie, 189
Pumpkin Pie Green Smoothie, 190
Snacks, 65–66, 149–150, 155
See also Small plates
Sodium, 128–129
Sofrito, 24, 197–198
Soups
Couscous Soup, 212–213
Hatz Lentil Soup, 213–214
Hearty Red Lentil Stew, 230–231
Hot, Sweet, and Sour *Bhamia* (Okra),
211–212
Potato Corn Chowder, 214
Sour Tofu Cream, 184
Soy
fatty acids in, 77 (table)
misunderstanding, 74–75
protein in, 97 (table)
See also Tempeh; Tofu
Spices, 108, 151, 172, 174
See also Flavors; *specific types of spices*
Spinach
carotenoids in, 117 (table)
Pumpkin Pie Green Smoothie, 190
Sports. *See* Athletes
Spreads. *See* Sauces and spreads
Sprinkles, 182–183
Sprouting, 105, 188
Squash. *See* Butternut squash; Zucchini
Staples
Basic Nut or Seed Milk, 176, 185
Betta' than Feta, 183
Bettermilk, 183–184
Date Paste, 184
DIY Nut or Seed Butter, 185–186
freezer, 160, 174–175
pantry, 160, 171–174
Parma Shake, 182
refrigerator, 160, 174, 182–186

Savory Sprinkles, 182–183
Sour Tofu Cream, 184
Starch, 72, 94, 103–105
    See also Grains
Stew, 230–231
Stone-Ground Cornbread, 216–217
Storage, 103, 170, 173–174
Stress, 26
Substitutions, 175–180
    dairy, 176–177, 182–185, 224–225
    egg, 177–178, 221–222, 223–224
    meat, 178–179
    oil, 179–180
Sugars. *See* Sweeteners
Summer Fruit Tart, 236
Sun therapy, 115
Sun-dried tomatoes
    Almond Sun-Dried Tomato Hummus, 193
    Savory Sprinkles, 182–183
Sunflower seeds
    Basic Seed Milk, 176, 185
    DIY Nut Butter, 185–186
Sunrise Kale Chips, 198–199
Supplements, 129–131
    for breastfeeding moms, 134
    for children, 137
    for infants, 134–135
    for pregnancy, 132–133
    for seniors, 138
Sustainability, 45–49
Sweeteners, 78–79, 179
    apricot paste, 196
    artificial, 79
    as carbohydrate type, 93–94
    Date Paste, 184
Synergy
    benefits and process, 22–24
    gut bacteria, 72
    nutritionism or, 62

Tabbouleh
    original recipe, 208
    Quinoa and Chickpea Tabbouleh Salad,
        208–209
Tahina, 191
Tapioca, 234
Tart, 236
Taylor, Henry, 9
Tea, 100, 126
    Moroccan Mint Chia Tea, 189–190
    Russian Tea Cookies, 235
    Vegiterranean Athlete's Drink, 190–191

Tempeh Cutlet Sandwich with Arugula and
    Basil Aioli, 220–221
TFAs. *See* Trans-fatty acids
Thiamin, 119
Thickeners, 106, 179
TMAO. *See* Trimethylamine *N*-oxide
Tofu
    benefits of, 74–75
    Betta' than Feta, 183
    Easy Caprese, 199–200
    egg replacement with, 178
    protein in, 97 (table)
    Shakshuka (Middle Eastern Tofu Scramble),
        223–224
    Sour Tofu Cream, 184
Tomatoes
    benefits of, 22, 24
    Fresh Tomato Dressing, 209–210
    Moussaka sauce, 233
    Sofrito, 24, 197–198
    See also Sun-dried tomatoes
Toxins
    in animal foods, 19–20, 36–38, 44
    BPA, 103
    in processed foods, 25
Trans-fatty acids (TFAs), 30, 31–32, 98–99
Traveling, 164–166
Trimethylamine *N*-oxide (TMAO), 20
Tuscan Garden Salad, 209–210

United States
    Cretan diet compared to, 7–8, 16–17
    Japanese diet compared to, 9–10
    protein intake in, 96
    sugar intake in, 78
Utensils, 169–170

Veganism. *See* Plant-based diet
Vegetables
    consumption increase in, 101–102
    dehydrating, 168–169
    egg replacement with, 178
    fatty acids in, 77 (table)
    fiber in, 72–73
    in food pyramids, 90 (fig.), 91 (fig.), 93
        (fig.), 100–102
    juicing, 168
    phytochemicals in, 68–69, 70 (table)
    Roasted Vegetable Sandwich Rolls, 219
    Savory Veggie Pancakes, 218
    selecting, viii, 102
    Simple Roasted Vegetables, 202–203

Vegetables (*continued*)
  See also Plant-based diet; *specific types of vegetables*
Vegiterranean Athlete's Drink, 190–191
Vegiterranean Diet
  for athletes, 138–139, 155–156, 190–191
  for breastfeeding moms, 134
  calorie consciousness tenet of, 80–83
  for children, 135–137, 154–155
  fats tenet of, 76–78
  fiber tenet of, 71–73
  for infants, 134–135
  inspiration for, ix–xi, 49–52, 57
  leafy greens tenet of, 75–76
  legumes tenet of, 73–75
  mindfulness tenet of, 85–86
  minerals in, 123–129
  movement tenet of, 83–85, 100
  packaging tenet of, 62–65
  for pregnancy, 132–133
  rainbow colors tenet of, 68–69, 70 (table)
  for seniors, 137–138
  simplicity tenet of, 65–67
  substitutions in, 175–180
  sweetener tenet of, 78–79
  tenets overview of, 61–62
  vitamins in, 115–122
  vitamins not in, 111–115
  water in, 93 (fig.), 100, 139
  for weight loss, 139–141
Vegiterranean Food Pyramid
  fats in, 105–107
  fruit and vegetables in, 100–102
  legumes in, 102–103
  overview, 91 (fig.), 92
  plate version of, 92–93, 93 (fig.)
  spices in, 108
  starches in, 103–105
  wine in, 108
Vegiterranean Meal Plan, 143–144
  for athletes, 155–156
  beverages, 150
  breakfast, 146–147, 153
  for children, 154–155
  condiments, 151
  desserts, 150
  for dining out, 161–166
  dinner, 148–149, 154
  lunch, 147–148, 154
  prepping, 160

  samples, 151–153
  snacks, 149–150
  tips, 144–146
Vinaigrette, 195–196
Vinegars, 108, 200, 238
Vitamin A, 116, 117 (table)
Vitamin B1, 119
Vitamin B2, 119–120
Vitamin B3, 120
Vitamin B5, 120–121
Vitamin B6, 121
Vitamin B7, 121
Vitamin B9, 121–122
Vitamin B12, 111–112, 113 (table)
Vitamin C, 21, 24, 118–119, 126–127
Vitamin D, 113–114
Vitamin E, 116–117
Vitamin K, 117–118
Vitamins, 110
  in Vegiterranean Diet, 115–122
  not in Vegiterranean Diet, 111–115
  See also Supplements

Walnuts
  Italian Wedding Cookies, 235
  protein in, 97 (table)
  tart crust, 236
Water
  dispensers, 169
  intake, 93 (fig.), 100, 139
Wedding Cookies, 235
Weight loss, 139–141
  artificial sweeteners and, 79
  calorie reduction and, 27–28, 80–83
  dietary fats and, 76, 106
  fad diets, 24, 62
  hunger tracking, 81–82, 159
  support, 141
Wheat meat, 179
White beans. *See* Cannellini beans
Whole foods, 21–22
  simplicity of, 65–66
  synergy of, 22–24, 62, 72
Whole: Rethinking the Science of Nutrition (Campbell), 63
Wine, 34–35, 91 (fig.), 93 (fig.), 108

Zest, 181
Zinc, 129
Zucchini, 202–203
Zuppe. See Soups